Say Good Bye to Ménière's Disease

Here's How to Make Your World Stop Spinning

Fourth Edition

Neil G. Bauman, Ph.D.

Integrity First Publications

Lynden, WA

http://IntegrityFirstPublications.com

Say Good Bye to Ménière's Disease
—Here's How to Make Your World Stop Spinning

Fourth Edition

Another **Integrity First** book in the series:

Everything You Wanted to Know About Your Hearing Loss But Were Afraid to Ask
(Because You Knew You Wouldn't Hear the Answers Anyway!)

ISBN 978-1-935939-22-1

Integrity First Publications
1013 Ridgeway Drive,
Lynden, WA 98264-1057
Phone: (360) 778-1266
FAX: (360) 389-5226
Email: info@IntegrityFirstPublications.com
Website: http://IntegrityFirstPublications.com

Printed in the United States of America

Warning—Disclaimer

This book is for your education and reference. It is neither a medical manual nor a guide to self-treatment for medical problems. Do not construe this book as giving personal medical advice or instruction. The author is not a medical doctor and neither prescribes treatment nor treats medical problems and does not intend that you attempt to do so either. If you suspect that you have a medical problem related to your ears, seek competent professional medical help. Use the information in this book to help you make informed decisions, not as a substitute for any treatment that your doctor may have prescribed for you.

The information and opinions expressed in this book are the result of careful research. They are believed to be accurate and sound, based on the best judgment available to the author. If you fail to consult appropriate health professionals, you assume the risk of any injuries. Neither Integrity First Publications, the Center for Hearing Loss Help, nor the author assumes any responsibility for damages or losses incurred as a result of using the information in this book, nor for any errors or omissions. It is the responsibility of each reader to exercise good judgment in using any information contained in this book.

Contents

About the Author

Neil G. Bauman, Ph.D., (Dr. Neil), is the founder and director of the Center for Hearing Loss Help. He is a hearing loss coping skills specialist, researcher, author and speaker on issues pertaining to hearing loss. No stranger to hearing loss himself, he has lived with a life-long severe hereditary hearing loss.

Dr. Neil did not let his hearing loss stop him from achieving what he wanted to do. He earned several degrees in fields ranging from forestry to ancient astronomy (Ph. D.) and theology (Th. D.) in addition to his extensive studies in fields related to hearing loss.

His mission is helping hard of hearing people understand and successfully cope with their hearing losses and other ear conditions. To this end, he provides education, support and counsel to hard of hearing people through personal contact, as well as through his books, articles, presentations and seminars.

Dr. Neil is the author of eleven books and more than nine hundred articles on hearing-loss related topics. (See the back of this book for a list of his books.) In addition, he is a dynamic speaker. His presentations are in demand throughout the USA and Canada.

You can reach him at:

Neil Bauman, Ph.D.
Center for Hearing Loss Help
1013 Ridgeway Drive
Lynden, WA 98264-1057
Phone: (360) 778-1266
FAX: (260) 389-5226
Email: neil@hearinglosshelp.com
Web site: http://hearinglosshelp.com

Preface

Ménière's disease is a stranger that one day suddenly invades your life—unwanted and unbidden to be sure—but there nevertheless. How you cope with this mysterious stranger is up to you.

For about 140 years, little was known about the basic cause of Ménière's disease and ways to effectively treat it. Thus, doctors and people with Ménière's disease developed a number of tricks and tips that helped numbers of people better cope with their Ménière's disease.

In the previous edition's preface I wrote,

> There are a number of things you and your doctors can do in order to hopefully help bring your Ménière's disease under some degree of control so that it doesn't completely take over your life. Some treatments work for some people, and others work for others. However, no one treatment seems to work for everybody. In fact, often you may find that what works best is to use a number of tips and treatments at the same time. You and your doctors have to find what specific things work best for you with your own "brand" of Ménière's disease.

However, this all went out the window beginning in 1999 when Dr. Michael Burcon serendipitously discovered the underlying cause of Ménière's disease. In the years since then, he has refined his treatment and now can eliminate or significantly help virtually every Ménière's sufferer that comes to him.

I came across him and his work in 2014 and began researching this to see if it was really true. The good news is that I am thoroughly convinced that this is a true breakthrough. Thus, I have made major changes in this edition to reflect this new information.

I also changed the title from *The Agony of Ménière's Disease* to *Say Good Bye to Ménière's Disease* to reflect the fact that now you have an excellent chance of getting rid of your Ménière's disease, rather than just hoping to relieve some of its more severe symptoms.

At the same time, I have left most of the previous information intact because it may be useful to those people that still have some residual effects from their years with Ménière's. It is also available for those people who choose not to avail themselves of the help that upper cervical spine chiropractors can give them in alleviating or eliminating their Ménière's disease symptoms, or for those who do not have access to such a chiropractor.

Apart from going to an experienced upper cervical spine chiropractor that has successfully treated numbers of Ménière's patients, I am not specifically recommending any of the treatments I mention in this book. I have sought out the most promising and effective solutions, and am simply bringing them to your attention for your consideration. What you do with this information is up to you. Try any of these treatments that "tickle your fancy". Ignore those that don't. The choice is yours.

I do not have Ménière's disease myself, so I cannot speak from personal experience. However, I do know many people with Ménière's disease. In this book, I have distilled the accumulated wisdom of both doctors/researchers that work with Ménière's disease, and the people that live with this affliction every day.

You can rest assured that if I ever get Ménière's disease, I will first have my upper cervical spine checked out by an experienced upper cervical spine specialist. Then, if necessary, I'll turn to the various other remedies listed in this book to work to bring it under control. I believe this approach would work wonders if I ever got Ménière's. I believe it will work wonders for yours too.

Neil Bauman, Ph.D.

Chapter 1

What Is Ménière's Disease?

To most people in the medical community, Ménière's (main-YAIRZ) disease is a mysterious condition—I say mysterious because although it has been known for more than 150 years, doctors still don't know what Ménière's disease really is.

You see, unlike a typical disease where doctors can define it and test to see if you have it or not, Ménière's disease is not a disease as such. Rather, it is a collection of symptoms. Thus, more correctly, they should call it Ménière's syndrome.

Furthermore, since doctor's can't "find" Ménière's disease—they can't put their finger on it and say, "here's your problem"—they diagnose Ménière's disease by the process of elimination. In other words, they rule out everything else that "looks" somewhat like Ménière's disease. After they have done this, they diagnose whatever remains as Ménière's disease. Thus, Ménière's disease is what doctors call an idiopathic disease from idiopathic causes.

Intractable Vertigo

Severe Ménière's disease (intractable vertigo) is one of the top three most difficult conditions with which a person can live. It ranks Number 2 on the list between intractable pain and intractable tinnitus.[1]

"Idiopathic" is just a fancy medical term that means "unknown". In short, doctors are saying they don't know what Ménière's disease is, don't know what causes it, and consequently, don't know how to effectively treat it. To them, it remains a mystery.

If you don't know what Ménière's disease is like, here's the 30-second "elevator" version. Ménière's disease consists of four symptoms that typically appear as a series of "attacks". A classic Ménière's attack includes a fluctuating hearing loss, vertigo (or feelings of dizziness/imbalance) and often accompanied by nausea and vomiting, tinnitus (a roaring, rushing, hissing or other sound in one of your ears) and a feeling of fullness in your affected ear. An attack can last from a few minutes to a few hours to a few days.

Morbus Ménière's

Many Ménière's sufferers, when on-line emailing or texting about Ménière's disease, colloquially use the abbreviation MM, rather than the official abbreviation for Ménière's disease (MD) like you might expect. MM is the abbreviation for the Latin *Morbus Meniere*—literally "the disease of Ménière", or Ménière's disease.

How Common Is Ménière's Disease?

There is considerable variation in the countries around the world as to the prevalence of Ménière's disease. For example, in the United States, the best estimates are that about 218 people per 100,000[2] (about 2 people per 1,000 or 0.2% of the population) have Ménière's disease. Based on this rate, about 621,000 people in the USA have Ménière's disease.[3]

In Canada, researchers estimate at least 180,000 people suffer from Ménière's disease (6 per 1,000).[4] Estimates around the world vary immensely and range from 0.2 to 7.5 per 1,000. Because of milder, unreported cases, the true figure may very well be double this.

The incidence of Ménière's disease varies by ethnic background too. For some reason Ménière's disease is reported more commonly in Britain and Sweden than elsewhere.[5] Part of this variation "likely results from the tendency of many physicians to lump all cases of recurrent vertigo into the category of Ménière's disease"[6] whether it is truly Ménière's disease or not.

Interestingly enough, one study in the USA revealed that 20 people per 1000 believe they have Ménière's disease—10 times higher than the best estimates (above). This suggests "that misdiagnosis is far more common than the correct diagnosis!"[7]

Most frequently, Ménière's disease develops in people between the ages of 30 and 50, but it can occur at any age.[8,9] On the whole, Ménière's disease attacks men and women with equal frequency.

What Is Ménière's Disease Like?

If you suffer from Ménière's disease, then you know just how horrible an experience these attacks can be. Following are three real-life examples to help you understand the severe trauma such people suffer through.

A Ménière's attack typically begins with one or more bouts of vertigo. Here is how it began with Boris. One day, when he was in his mid-thirties, the room he was in suddenly began to spin. He quickly sat down and gripped the arms of the chair to steady himself while waves of nausea swept over him.

As the vertigo passed, he heard a persistent roaring in his left ear. In addition, he realized he couldn't hear as well as he used to. He was worried because the noise in his ear went on for two weeks. When he had two more similar episodes that year, Boris began to worry he had a brain tumor. He became fearful that an attack would begin at some awkward moment and possibly jeopardize his life. His former confidence gave way to constant anxiety.[10]

Classic Ménière's Symptoms

In 1861, Dr. Prosper Ménière wrote a classic description of the condition that now bears his name.

"A man, young and robust, suddenly, without apparent reason, experienced vertigo, nausea and vomiting. He was in a state of inexpressible anguish and prostration. His face was pale and bathed in sweat as if about to faint. Often the patient, after seeming to stagger in a dazed state, fell to the ground unable to get up. Lying on his back, he could not open his eyes without his environment becoming as a whirlpool. The smallest movements of his head worsened his feeling of vertigo and nausea."[11]

To Muriel, Ménière's disease is a dreaded, disabling affliction. Depending on the severity of her attacks, she experiences mild to violent dizziness/vertigo. During light attacks she may be able to manage on unsteady legs—bumping into door jambs or furniture—trying to carry out necessary chores around the house. Severe attacks are another story. At such times she has no sense of balance whatsoever. She can't walk or otherwise move around. Her overwhelming sensation is the horrendous spinning of the world around her and the attending nausea.[12]

Mark has constant severe disequilibrium. He explained,

> I used to have terrible vertigo attacks. The room would spin in one direction constantly for a week or two, then in the opposite direction for "daze" on end. Then it would stop for a week, or several months, and then start again.

Normally, Ménière's disease only occurs in one ear, at least initially, although about 10% of the people getting Ménière's disease have it in both ears from the outset.[13] However, about 20 to 25 percent, (although some experts report up to 50 percent[14,15,16]) of Ménière's sufferers find that it later develops in their other ear, usually within 2 or 3 years.[17,18]

According to one researcher, 75% of the people who will ultimately get Ménière's disease in both ears will have done so within 5 years.[19] By the time people have had Ménière's disease for 30 years, about 50% of them will have it in both ears.[20] The good news is that you still have a 50 to 80 percent chance that your Ménière's will never affect your other ear!

One person asked, "When a person begins experiencing Ménière's symptoms, do they hit all at once or gradually?"

While full-blown Ménière's attacks may occur without warning, many Ménière's sufferers experience a feeling of fullness in one ear for several hours or days preceding the attack. Also, tinnitus often occurs, or increases, just before an attack. Another common sign of an impending attack is a drop in hearing.

Here is how one lady described the onset of her attacks.

> My symptoms do not happen all at once. Sometimes I have strong vertigo attacks for 10 to 15 minutes, and then nausea will hit. Sometimes, in between the vertigo attacks, the tinnitus starts. Each Ménière's attack is different for me. After 35 years of experiencing them, no two have been the same.

Julie noted, "Both of my severe attacks came on without any warning at all."

Alan explained,

> My vertigo attacks were surrounded by a sort of fog of disequilibrium. Often I could tell when an attack was coming a few hours before it hit me because things just were "off". My vision seemed to lag behind my movements; I was unsteady; my hearing decreased; and my tinnitus increased.

The frequency of Ménière's attacks are unpredictable. Typically you will get one or more attacks a year. Then, again, you may have a single attack and never have another one, or you may have another bout five years later. Often, Ménière's attacks may come in clusters. For example, you might have a number of attacks all in one week, and then might not have another attack for weeks, months or even years. If you are particularly unfortunate, you may have daily or monthly attacks occurring over a period of years.

A Ménière's attack may be mild, and over in a few minutes, or may last for up to 24 hours. The onset of these attacks is frequently quite sudden—reaching peak intensity within minutes—and lasting for an hour or more before subsiding. You may just feel that you are about to be dizzy. Or you may have a brief, mild attack of dizziness. Then again, you may have continuous, mild dizziness that goes on for hours, days or weeks.

The Four Symptoms of Classic Ménière's Disease

A full-blown Ménière's attack includes the following four symptoms.

Vertigo

First, there are periodic attacks of vertigo (where the room seems to spin around, or you spin around and the room stays still). The vertigo from Ménière's attacks is unlike any vertigo people without Ménière's have ever experienced. Alan described his vertigo attacks this way.

> The vertigo gave me the sensation of the world spinning around me. With my right ear, the spinning seemed to go from left to right. Later, when my left ear got Ménière's, I felt sort of a forward-spinning sensation. This was harder to deal with in terms of remaining on my feet.

Vertigo is the main, and most distressing, symptom of Ménière's disease. Alan further explained,

> Vertigo is the most devastating part of Ménière's attacks. I have Ménière's as severely as anyone I've ever heard of. It's in both my ears. In the beginning, I could sense an impending vertigo attack as much as a couple of days before it came on. My hearing level would drop, and the tinnitus would increase dramatically. Then I'd have a vertigo episode that would last anywhere from 4 to 24 hours. I'd be flat on my back with the world whirling around. Medications didn't help. It got so that I was having them maybe once every 7 to 8 days.

Vertigo vs. Dizziness

Dizziness is the feeling of being giddy or unsteady, and produces a sensation of imbalance. Vertigo, on the other hand, is the perception of spinning. You perceive the world is spinning around you, or that you are spinning yourself.

The sensation of spinning typically also produces nystagmus (an involuntary rapid movement of the eyes from side to side)

In order to cope, I'd try to squeeze in as much as I could get done in between attacks.

This vertigo may be disabling enough to force you to lie down. Some people have such severe attacks that they suddenly drop to the floor as if they had been pole-axed. These "drop attacks" leave you totally helpless as your world spins, and you vomit severely.

Drop Attacks—Otolithic Crisis of Tumarkin

The fancy name for drop attacks is "otolithic crisis of Tumarkin". There are a number of causes of drop attacks. Approximately 5% are due to Ménière's disease.[22]

Leigh has experienced a number of drop attacks. As she explains,

> A drop attack is when you are literally thrown to the ground quite violently with a severe case of spinning vertigo. I've blacked out from the force of hitting my head either on the way down or when I hit the ground. You cannot get your hands out in time and that's the scariest part of it. I've hit my head many times and opened it up a few times.

Mary recounted,

> I was out jogging with my dog. I don't know what happened other than at one point I felt real dizzy and unable to get my bearings straight. At that point I fell headfirst to the ground. When I came to, my husband said he saw me bounce when my head hit. I ended up with a concussion and cracked ribs. I have never had Ménière's hit me instantly like that before. I mostly feel dizzy before I fall, but this time there was no warning at all.

Ménière's attacks don't necessarily start out being drop attacks. As Alan explained,

> Mine didn't start until my second ear became involved. At some point, I no longer got the few hours of disequilibrium and warning before the vertigo occurred. It would happen suddenly without warning.

Alan added,

> When my right ear went bad, the vertigo sensation was horizontal—as if I was standing at the center of a merry-go-round. When my left ear went bad, the vertigo from the drop attacks was often, though not always, a vertical sensation—as if I was suddenly rolled forwards. Not fun!

Linda had a "funny" drop attack experience. She explains,

> I went out for a walk today. About half a block from home, I suddenly slowed down because although my legs were going forward, it felt like

someone (or some force) was pushing my upper body backward, and I lost my balance.

"Cindy" reported,

In my attacks, I would go from feeling absolutely no warning (a couple times. I was just walking through my home) and then "Bam!" I would suddenly feel like I was almost pushed into the carpet. It was not like falling, but more like one second I was walking and the next second I was slamming my face into the carpet. It made me very hesitant to do things like get on a ladder, or stand next to the edge of an embankment, that sort of thing. I did not lose consciousness, but it almost felt like there was a gap in time between walking along and hitting the ground with a "bounce".

"Sally" explained,

My drop attacks had been happening at home for months. I had many bruises, but I was in denial and just made some excuse, picked myself up and went on. Then it happened at work. One minute I was up right at the water cooler and the next thing I remember I was staring up from the floor with my boss standing over me asking what happened. All I could tell him was that I was standing one minute and the next it was like I was a puppet with my strings cut. My knees just disappeared out from under me and I crumpled to the ground, hitting hard on the way down. I couldn't trust myself not to suddenly end up "ass over teakettle". That expression very much captures my feelings of, "What? How did I get down here?" and "Ouch!" "What did I hit on the way down?" This is one of the shocking things about drop attacks.

These attacks can be over in just a few minutes or go on for hours. Some people with Ménière's disease get these drop attacks frequently, others only every year or two. Fortunately, many never get them.[21]

After Ménière's attacks you will likely be tired (or exhausted if it was a bad attack) and will want to sleep for hours (or even days). As one lady explained,

Some Ménière's attacks are more severe than others—requiring my sleeping them off anywhere from 1 hour to 16 hours.

Until you get to know your condition, if you had a mild attack, you might think you just had a badly upset stomach.[23] Even after the vertigo passes, the feelings of unsteadiness and imbalance may linger for days. Fortunately, many people are symptom-free between their attacks, while other people experience varying degrees of mild imbalance, hearing loss and tinnitus between attacks. Fortunately, the symptoms of Ménière's disease tend to disappear over time.[24]

For many people with Ménière's disease, vertigo is the worst symptom, and is the symptom with which they have the most trouble coping. Vertigo can totally incapacitate you. It disrupts virtually every aspect of your life since you can't move without getting sick. The associated nausea, sweating and vomiting are classic symptoms of motion sickness.

As Dr. Hazell dryly notes,

> Lying on the floor in a public place, being sick, does not always bring out the most charitable feelings in other people![25]

Pam graphically pictured her severe Ménière's attacks this way.

> I was ending up in the emergency room for a day every 3 to 4 weeks—barfing my brains out, and heaving for hours when there was nothing left to barf!

Less severe Ménière's attacks can still disrupt your life. For example, Julie related,

> I think my car is moving when it's not. When I am a passenger in a car on long trips, I can't read, I can't work on my laptop computer, nothing. My eyes just won't focus on the task I'm trying to do. I get disoriented with trying to read or concentrate on anything visual. As a result, I end up getting lots of sleep!

"Andy" reported,

> After the attack is over, I have bad balance and feelings of queasiness for the next day or two.

This is Leigh's experience too. She explained,

> After an attack, the feeling of being unbalanced continues—so does the queasiness. If it's a bad one, sometimes taking Meclizine helps me.

Tinnitus

The second symptom of a full-blown Ménière's attack is tinnitus. Tinnitus from Ménière's disease is typically a low-pitched incessant hissing,[26] rushing or roaring noise rather than a high-pitched sound.[27] Your tinnitus may persist, fluctuate or disappear between attacks.

Coping with Your Tinnitus

You can learn more about tinnitus and how to deal with it in our comprehensive companion book, *Take Control of Your Tinnitus—Here's How.* (See the back of this book for further details.)

Hearing Loss

The third Ménière's symptom is a fluctuating sensorineural hearing loss, typically first showing up in the lower frequencies.[28] Thus, your audiogram will often reveal a mild or moderate reverse-slope (low-frequency) hearing loss. As Ménière's disease progresses, it will typically affect all frequencies of sound.

Hearing usually improves between attacks, but it often worsens with each succeeding attack. Thus, you may experience a step-wise hearing loss—two steps down, one step back up. Your hearing loss may eventually dip to severe or profound[29] at all frequencies. Fortunately, it seldom results in total hearing loss.

As well as having difficulty hearing, music and voices may now sound tinny or distorted. Loud sounds may become abnormally loud. Also, the fluctuating hearing loss may make wearing hearing aids difficult. As Margo says,

> I have good days and bad days. Even I don't know how well I will hear when I wake up, or even 30 minutes from now.

Feeling of Fullness

The fourth and final symptom of full-blown Ménière's disease is a feeling of fullness or pressure in your ear or head. Your ear probably feels "plugged" like you have come down a long hill and need to swallow to clear the pressure. However, swallowing will not clear this feeling of pressure because your Eustachian tube is not working properly at this point.

Some people experience this feeling of fullness in slightly different ways. For example, when James has a Ménière's attack, the severe pressure in his head makes him feel like his head is under water.

After an attack, you slowly recover. Your vertigo goes away; your tinnitus and the feelings of pressure in your ear usually disappear; and your hearing tends to return to a new "normal" near, but below, its previous level. Alan recounted,

> After a vertigo attack, my tinnitus and hearing generally improved, but I'd still have a period of disequilibrium. There definitely was a recovery period and sleep helped.

Symptoms That May Accompany Ménière's Disease

Although Ménière's disease, as defined, only has the above four symptoms, a number of secondary symptoms may accompany your Ménière's attacks. In addition, still other symptoms may reveal themselves between attacks. Here are some of them.

Emotional problems: Damage to your vestibular system can include emotional problems such as anxiety, frustration, anger and depression. Your feelings of self-confidence and self-esteem may plummet. You may feel vaguely uneasy. You may feel that something is wrong or unreal without knowing why.

Anxiety: Since your Ménière's attacks may appear at random, and at the most inopportune times at that, you may suffer from anxiety—worrying that you may have a Ménière's attack when you are out. In extreme cases, you may let your anxiety keep you housebound.

Depression: If the treatments you try are not successful, and if you perceive that you are "stuck" with this horrible Ménière's disease for the rest of your life, you may become depressed. You may also be depressed because you can no longer do certain activities you once enjoyed.

Brain fog (Memory problems): Unlikely as it seems, vestibular damage from Ménière's can cause brain fog and memory problems. Here is why. When your Ménière's disease has seriously damaged your balance system, keeping your balance is now largely a conscious effort, not the automatic effortless procedure it once was. You now have to expend a lot of brain power to consciously do things to keep your balance. Consequently, those areas of your brain that you once just used for thought and memory, now must constantly work on keeping you balanced. As a result, your memory may suffer. You may grope for words when talking. You may easily forget what is being spoken about during a conversation. You may be easily distracted. You may have difficulty comprehending directions or instructions. You may have trouble concentrating and may feel disoriented at times. In short, you feel as though your brain is "fogged in".

Fatigue: Severe attacks of vertigo may leave you so drained and exhausted that you sleep for hours afterwards. Furthermore, if your balance system is damaged, you now have to consciously work hard to keep yourself erect. All this work makes you tired! Thus, you may suffer from chronic fatigue.

Muscular aches and pains: Vestibular damage due to Ménière's may also give rise to muscular aches and pains. This is because you now have to consciously control your balance by making your muscles rigid and less relaxed as you strain to keep your balance. In addition, you may get headaches and a stiff/sore neck from trying to hold your head absolutely still so you won't feel dizzy or nauseous.

Recruitment & Hyperacusis: As a result of hearing loss caused by Ménière's attacks, you may find that certain everyday sounds are now too loud for you. You may even perceive them as so loud that they hurt.

Recruitment is a byproduct of a sensorineural hearing loss (the same kind of hearing loss that Ménière's disease causes). You may find that tinkling cutlery, dishes clattering, the dog barking or a door slamming now seem to "blow the top of your head off" whereas these sounds did not bother you before.

Hyperacusis occurs from damage to the auditory system. You now perceive many/most/all normal sounds as too loud. It's as though your brain's internal volume control is stuck on "high".

Whether you have recruitment or hyperacusis (or both), the result is the same—you perceive normal everyday sounds as being too loud to stand.

Migraine headaches: Migraine headaches and Ménière's attacks often go together since migraine headaches and Ménière's attacks can both arise from the same underlying cause.

You may also get a different kind of migraine, called a vestibular migraine. Rather than having a standard migraine headache, you get pain in your ear. As Mary explained,

> I was diagnosed with vestibular migraines. My doctor was surprised I don't have headaches, but when I described the pain he said, "Ah! Headaches in the ear!" That is exactly how I would describe this feeling.

Nystagmus: (nye-STAG-muss) During a Ménière's attack, you may also experience nystagmus. This is a secondary result of severe vertigo resulting from a damaged vestibular (balance) system. Nystagmus develops if your vestibular system is only damaged on one side or damaged worse on one side than the other.

Nystagmus refers to abnormal rapid rhythmic back-and-forth side-to-side involuntary eye movements (eye jerking). With nystagmus, both of your eyes drift slowly in one direction and then suddenly jerk in the opposite direction. Your eyes will jerk toward the undamaged (less damaged) side and will drift back towards the (more) damaged side. This abnormal eye movement can also cause vertigo, nausea, vomiting and a host of other visual complaints.

"The dizzies": You may have "the dizzies", which is really just very mild vertigo. You may experience "the dizzies" for hours, days or weeks after a Ménière's attack. You don't feel you are spinning as you would during a severe Ménière's attack, but you definitely feel "off balance". Alan described this feeling of disequilibrium or feeling of being off balance thus.

> When you move your head or body, you feel as though you are out of sync with your surroundings. Maybe the floor feels as if it's not quite level, or as if you are on a gently rocking ship.

How Ménière's Disease May Progress

The natural progression of Ménière's disease varies from person to person. The symptoms of Ménière's disease change over time—more slowly in some, and more quickly in others. About 70% of the people with Ménière's disease find their vertigo attacks diminish over time—with or without medical intervention. The other 30% of people with Ménière's disease experience unrelenting vertigo and thus may choose aggressive invasive medical therapy.[30]

In severe cases, initially you may have between 3 and 10 attacks per month. However, after two years, you have a 50% chance that you will not have any more episodes. If you do, you will likely have less than 3 attacks per month. After 8 years, you only have a relatively slight chance of having any more attacks. Unfortunately, a few people still have some Ménière's attacks for several more decades, but normally fewer than 3 a month.[31]

Ménière's disease may progress through three stages. Not everyone experiences all three of these stages. Furthermore, everyone progresses through these stages at their own rate. It is highly variable.

Stage One

In the beginning, here is the way Ménière's disease typically acts. You experience sudden attacks of vertigo that can last from 15 or 20 minutes upward to several hours. In this stage, your attacks of vertigo usually cause nausea and vomiting, as well as other motion-sickness-like symptoms such as sweating and cold, clammy skin. At this point, even slight head movements can aggravate your vertigo and cause further vomiting.

Rather than getting someone to rush you to the hospital (a common reaction), Dr. Gibson suggests that it is better to lie down in bed, possibly take an anti-emetic drug and wait for the vertigo attack to pass.[32]

In this stage, all you can think about is your terrible vertigo. You may be completely unaware of any hearing loss (or distorted hearing), tinnitus or feelings of fullness in your ear that may be occurring at the same time. After such an attack, your ear returns to normal (or near normal). Thus, when you see an ear specialist, he can't find anything wrong.

About 50% of people with Stage 1 Ménière's disease can expect their Ménière's to go into remission. Your remission may be permanent, or it may last for a number of years, even after several clusters of attacks.[33]

Stage Two

By the time your Ménière's reaches Stage 2, you will have permanent hearing loss and tinnitus. Your hearing will no longer bounce back to normal after each attack, but will partially recover to a "new normal".

With each attack, your hearing fluctuates, along with your tinnitus and the feeling of fullness in your ear. In this stage, these fluctuations in hearing, tinnitus and/or feelings of fullness in your ear may warn you that another Ménière's attack is imminent.

Your Ménière's attacks will often tend to occur in clusters that can last for several months. Fortunately, by this time, you likely will have learned to manage your vertigo so you don't vomit much anymore, and you may find that you still experience long periods of remission between your Ménière's attacks.

You may remain in Stage 2 and never progress to Stage 3. Actually, only about 50% of people in this stage ever progress to Stage 3.[34]

Stage Three

This final stage of Ménière's disease is sometimes called the "burnt-out" stage (although current thinking is that Ménière's disease does not ever really "burn out"). A better term is "late-stage" Ménière's disease. You may never reach this stage.

In Stage 3, your hearing usually reaches a very low level and no longer fluctuates. Your hearing may be so bad that hearing aids don't significantly help you. If this is the case, and you have Ménière's disease in both ears, you may choose to get cochlear implants in order to hear again. Although you will still have your tinnitus, by this time you may have become habituated to your tinnitus so it no longer really bothers you.

You may find that you no longer have vertigo attacks, or that they are now quite mild compared to what they used to be. Thus, you may no longer need to take any medications. George explained,

> I have had Ménière's disease for over 17 years. Back when my Ménière's cycle was at its highest, all of the triggers worked against me. I had to double all my medications. Now I don't take any medications. My otolaryngologist finally took me off the diuretics and *Valium.*

In Stage 3, your balance system is now basically destroyed in the ear with your Ménière's. As a result, you have poor overall balance.[35] Attacks of vertigo may be replaced by more constant struggles with vision and balance, including difficulty walking in the dark, and occasional sudden loss of balance.[36] Also, sometimes drop attacks of vestibular origin occur in this stage. If you have Ménière's disease in both ears, you may be left with basically no balance at all.

Pattern of Hearing Loss as Ménière's Disease Progresses

In the beginning (Stage 1), your hearing loss will likely show a low-frequency hearing loss (Fig. 1-1), often called a reverse-slope loss from the shape of the audiogram (sloping **up** to the right—rather than the typical audiogram which shows hearing loss sloping **down** to the right). Initially hearing loss in the low frequencies may be 40 or 50 dB, rising to normal or near normal by about 1,000 Hz or so.

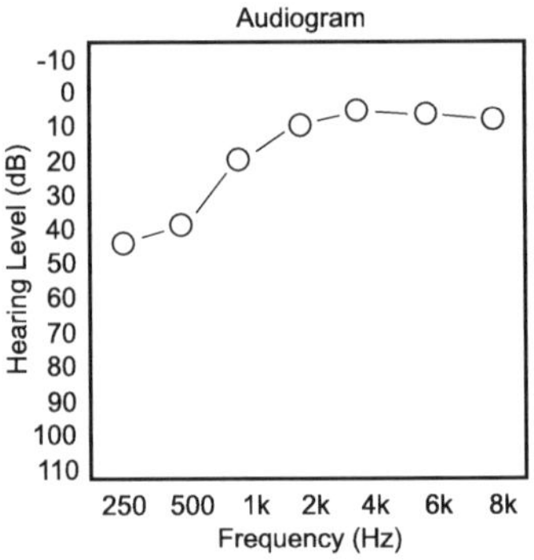

Fig. 1-1. Typical audiogram of a person in Stage 1 of Ménière's disease showing a reverse-slope (low-frequency) hearing loss.

As your Ménière's disease progresses (Stage 2), it may begin to affect your high frequencies also. At this point, your audiogram may have a reverse cookie-bite loss shape—high in the middle and low at each end—as though someone had taken a bite out of the bottom of your audiogram (Fig. 1-2). Your overall hearing loss will likely be moderate at this point—perhaps in the 40 to 60 dB range.

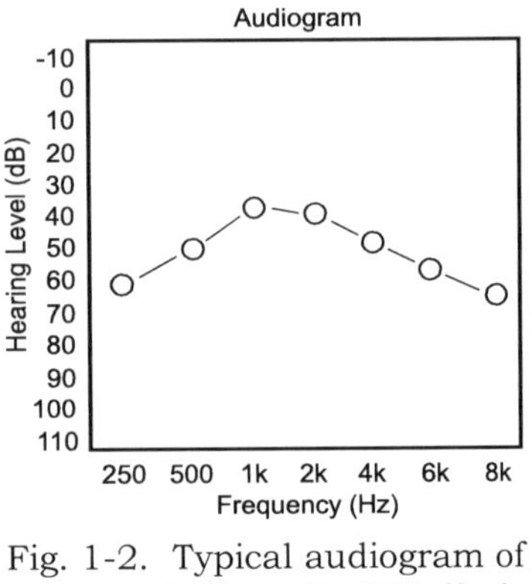

Fig. 1-2. Typical audiogram of a person in Stage 2 of Ménière's disease showing a reverse cookie-bite hearing loss (greater hearing loss in both the low and high frequencies).

As you reach Stage 3, your audiogram may become more of a flat line—what they call a "flat curve"—in the severe to profound range (Fig. 1-3). Your audiogram may reveal a hearing loss of perhaps 70 to 90 dB or greater.

Of course, there can be tremendous variability to the above, but this gives you an idea of how, on the average, hearing loss due to Ménière's disease may progress.

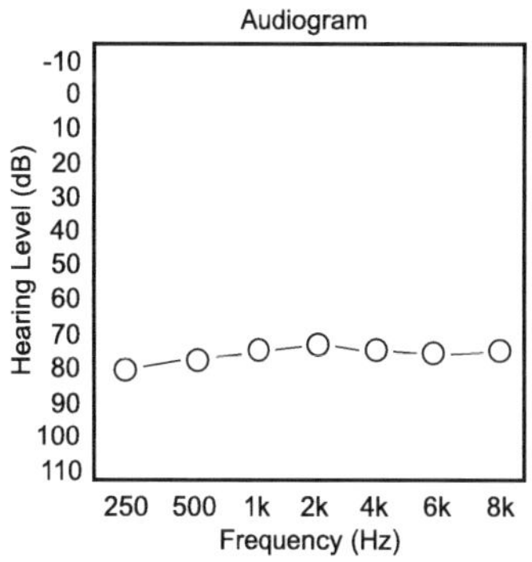

Fig. 1-3. Typical audiogram of a person with late-stage (Stage 3) Ménière's disease showing a more or less flat curve bordering on a severe to profound hearing loss.

Chapter 1 Endnotes

1 Hogan, 1998. p. 61.
2 Gates, 2004. p. 718.
3 Hain, 2009a. p. 1.
4 Engel, 1993. p. 160.
5 Salt, 1998a. p. 2.
6 Hain, 2009a. p. 1.
7 Hain, 2011a. p. 3.
8 Ménière's Disease, 1997. p. 2.
9 Vernick, 1993. p. 172.
10 Engel, 1993. pp. 160-161.
11 Hazell, 1982.
12 Adey, 1989.
13 Gibson, 2003. p. 2.
14 Hain, 2009a. p. 1.
15 Hain, 2011a. p. 2.
16 Gibson, 2003. p. 2.
17 Ménière's Disease, 1997. p. 5.
18 Vernick, 1993. p. 173.
19 Hain, 2011a. p. 2.
20 Hain, 2011a. p. 2.
21 Hines, 1997. p 3.
22 Hain, 2009b. p. 1.
23 Engel, 1993. pp. 161.
24 Vernick, 1993. p. 173.
25 Hazell, 1982.
26 Hazell, 1982.
27 Vernick, 1993. p. 172.
28 Hazell, 1982.
29 Vernick, 1993. p. 173.
30 Gates, 2004. p. 718.
31 Salt, 1998a. p. 3.
32 Gibson, 2003. p. 1.
33 Gibson, 2003. p. 1.
34 Gibson, 2003. p. 1.
35 Gibson, 2003. p. 1.
36 Ménière's Disease, 2010. p. 1.

Chapter 2

Ménière's Disease and Your Balance System

A lady wrote,

> I've read that eventually the balance system is irreversibly damaged in most people with Ménière's disease. I was wondering how people cope with mobility at this point. Is a cane or walker still helpful, or does it mean a wheelchair? What do most people do?

Ménière's disease can indeed damage the balance system in your ears. However, even totally destroying this balance system (doctors call it the vestibular system) doesn't relegate you to a wheelchair. Let me explain.

Our ears are incredibly complex organs. Many people just think of them as their means of hearing, but they are, at the same time, our primary organs of balance.

Perhaps you weren't aware of this, but your vestibular system does not work alone to maintain your balance. When God designed your body, He gave you not just one, not just two, but **three** separate, yet interconnected, balance systems. That way, if anything went wrong with one system, you would not be totally without balance, and left to flop helplessly on the floor like a jellyfish.

Your Three Balance Systems

The major component regulating your balance is, of course, the vestibular system in your inner ears. Your vestibular system consists of the three semicircular canals, the saccule and the utricle. This part of your inner ear continuously senses gravity and both straight and curved movement. Like the cochlea, the vestibular structures contain thousands of tiny hair cells that generate and relay balance signals to your brain.[1]

As you likely know, if something damages the hair cells in your cochlea, you end up with hearing problems. Likewise, if something damages the hair cells in your vestibular system, the result is balance problems.

The second component of your balance system is your eyes (ocular system). Your eyes see both your position in space and movement.

The final component of your balance system goes by the tongue-twisting name of proprioceptive (proh-pree-oh-SEP-tiv) system. Your proprioceptive system uses special pressure sensors in your muscles, tendons and joints to sense gravity and joint position. Most of your proprioceptive sensors are in your feet and leg joints.

As long as these three systems are working properly, you seldom give your ability to keep your balance any thought. However, if one or more of these systems ever fails, it can impose enormous changes on your lifestyle.

These three systems cooperate closely with each other in an interdependent manner to use the strengths of each to the best advantage.

Your Ears and Eyes Work Together

Your vestibular system works together with your eyes in what doctors call the vestibulo-ocular reflex. What this reflex accomplishes is truly incredible. When you walk, your head moves up and down with your body movement. This would make everything you see blurry unless you were absolutely still. However, your vestibulo-ocular reflex normally keeps your eyes clearly focused on your surroundings by instantly and continuously changing your eye position as you move. You think nothing of this. It is totally subconscious and automatic.

However, if your eyes and ears lose this coordination due to vestibular damage, your eye muscles do not receive the proper signals from your brain to automatically adjust for this movement. As a result, your surroundings will appear to move, bounce, jiggle and jump about and your vision will be blurry. This means you will find driving extremely difficult. You will also find it very difficult to read signs as you walk. Some people can't even recognize the faces of the people they see walking towards them on the sidewalk. The technical name for this condition is oscillopsia (ah-sih-LOP-see-ah).

Alan explains,

> At first, oscillopsia can be fairly severe and bothersome, but over time, your brain adjusts and it becomes less of a problem. Now that both of my ears are out of commission, my oscillopsia is permanent, but not as severe as it was at first. I don't really notice it unless I'm in motion while trying to see something in detail at a distance, such as a sign, or trying to do something like read a map while bouncing along in a car.

If you have oscillopsia, just walking can be extremely difficult because it is difficult to see and respond to obstacles in your path and to sense the exact location of the floor or ground.

Your vestibulo-ocular reflex is so sensitive that it actually senses the tiny upward and downward motions your head makes each time you breathe in and out. It sends this information to your brain. Your brain, in turn, instructs your eye muscles to keep your eyes clearly focused on what you are doing in spite of this movement.

Even more astounding is how incredibly sensitive your vestibulo-ocular reflex is. In fact, it is so incredibly sensitive that it detects the miniscule movement and change in position of your head each time your heart beats and relays this information to your brain. Again, your brain sends messages to your eye muscles to correct for this, all unknown to you. By doing so, it reduces the movement of the image on your retinas thus giving you clear vision so you can read fine print and see fine detail. If you are like most people, you probably never had an inkling that day after day your ears were doing this amazing job for you.

You need your eyes to help you maintain your balance. At the same time, you need your ears (vestibular system) to help you maintain clear vision. Anything that disrupts your vestibulo-ocular reflex directly affects your vision. Therefore, if your vestibular system is damaged, you will likely have fuzzy or blurred vision. You will also likely have difficulty focusing on objects or holding your eyes on a printed page since your hands can't hold a book completely steady. (Each heartbeat not only "jerks" your head, but also "jerks" your hands a tiny bit too.) This makes it difficult or impossible to read smaller print. It can also make it difficult to write. At the same, you will probably have difficulty with depth perception and focusing on or watching moving objects.

In addition, you may feel dizzy, experience nausea or have a sense of moving, particularly at the onset, if you move your eyes, move your head and eyes simultaneously, or watch moving objects. This can make being around traffic, riding in a vehicle, watching TV or watching a movie in a movie theater very unpleasant. You may find moving or flickering lights bother you.

Just the act of focusing your eyes may be difficult and can lead to dizziness and nausea. You may have a tendency to look down because it is harder to focus on more distant objects. Your ability to accurately determine distances may also be disrupted. As a result of your poor depth perception, you may often bump into things.

Your Ears and Proprioceptive System Work Together

Your vestibular system also works together with the muscles of your body via your spinal cord in what doctors call the vestibulo-spinal reflex. This instantaneous reflex allows for continual, coordinated muscle adjustments so you can maintain your balance as you change position.

Normally, your vestibular system sends balance information to those areas of your brain and nervous system involved in the motor control of your muscles. This balance information allows your brain to continuously make little adjustments in muscle activity and body position to allow you to stand upright and maintain your balance.

When you lose this reflex, your vestibular system no longer passes this information on to your brain or it passes faulty information. As a result, your brain does not order the tiny muscle adjustments and you get a condition known as ataxia (ah-TAKS-see-ah). Ataxia is the inability to coordinate your muscles properly such that it affects your gait. As a result, when you walk you may lurch and stagger as if you were drunk (staggering gait) as the other two parts of your balance system try to compensate. You will be unsteady and stumble a lot.

You may try to compensate for this by standing and walking with your legs farther apart than normal in order to give you better control of your balance (wide-based gait). You also may keep looking down while you are walking. Even so, you may lose your balance or stagger when turning quickly (whole body or head only), and need to hold on to walls or furniture when you are walking.

In addition, you may have difficulty walking on slippery, soft or slanted surfaces or on uneven ground. You may have difficulty standing or walking in dim or dark places, at night, or when you have your eyes closed. As Alan explains,

> For me walking in the dark is hard, and it's even worse if there are moving lights in my visual field. That could include headlights from cars, moving lights on signs, or even from a flashlight I'm carrying.

Even under good lighting conditions, you will still tend to stagger. You may also feel unsteady, have problems standing with your feet together, be uncoordinated and clumsy and overreach when grabbing for objects.

Two Systems Are Necessary to Maintain Balance

When they are working properly, your brain uses the separate signals from your vestibular, ocular and proprioceptive systems to instantly and subconsciously maintain clear vision and to make rapid muscle adjustments to maintain your balance and prevent you from falling.

These three systems are somewhat redundant, so if one stops functioning, you can manage (with difficulty) on the remaining two. However, you cannot maintain your balance with just one system working—you need at least two and preferably all three. Since your vestibular system is your major balance system, if you lose it, your brain has to rely on the other two systems. However, without the critical vestibular information, you will have much more trouble maintaining your balance, especially in the dark since darkness effectively eliminates your ocular system leaving you with just your proprioceptive system to help you.

When Damage Wrecks Your Balance System

So far we have been looking at how the vestibular system works together with the other two systems and what can happen when the vestibular system totally ceases to function. However, often the vestibular system is just damaged, not totally destroyed. This gives rise to a whole new set of problems.

When your vestibular system dies, it no longer sends any information to your brain, so your brain does the best it can with the information from the other two systems.

However, if your vestibular system is only damaged such as often happens with Ménière's disease, especially in the initial stages, it continues to send balance information—wrong information, mind you—but your brain doesn't know this. This confuses your brain and you will experience things such as dizziness and vertigo (VER-tih-goe). If you have vertigo, you may feel that you are spinning around or the room you are in is spinning around you.

Vertigo results from a mismatch of vestibular, ocular, and proprioceptive inputs. When all three are telling your brain the same thing, all is well. However, when your ears tell your brain one thing and your eyes and proprioceptive system tell it another thing, your brain doesn't know which to believe. In this case, your brain's confusion manifests itself as vertigo. Nausea and vomiting often accompany vertigo.

Vestibular side effects generally are worse in the first few weeks after vestibular damage occurs. In time, your brain will begin to rely less and less on vestibular information and more and more on ocular and proprioceptive inputs. As this happens the dizziness and vertigo (with the attendant nausea and vomiting) will tend to go away and you will tend to function as though your vestibular system were completely dead. However, you will be left with permanent side effects that can alter your lifestyle dramatically.

When Your Balance System Is Not Running on All Six Cylinders

As we have seen, we have three separate, but interconnected, balance systems, our ears, our eyes and our proprioceptive systems. This gives us some built-in redundancy in case one system is damaged.

Not only that, but each of these three separate systems consist of two (redundant) subsystems. For example, you have a separate vestibular (balance) system in **each** of your inner ears. Whenever one side is damaged or destroyed, the other side takes over and allows you to keep your balance.

Thus, your balance system actually consists of six separate parts. Think of it as a six cylinder motor. When all of the six cylinders are working together properly, the motor just purrs along. However, if one or more cylinders quits working, your car motor begins missing and running very rough, just like what happens when you lose one or more parts of your "6-cylinder" balance system.

However, unlike in a car motor, the cylinders of your balance system are not all the same size. Your balance system "motor" consists of two large cylinders (your vestibular system), two medium-sized cylinders (your ocular system) and two small cylinders (your proprioceptive system).

Thus, most of your balance "horsepower" is generated from the two big vestibular cylinders. When one goes, it leaves a big hole in your balance system, but the motor still runs. However, now your balance system is weaker and you have balance issues, especially under difficult balance conditions.

This is exactly what happens to the vast majority of people with Ménière's disease. Since Ménière's disease typically only attacks one ear (one large cylinder), you still have some balance function. Thus, most people with Ménière's, unless they are having a severe vertigo attack where they can't even sit up, use whatever balance systems (cylinders) are still working and manage to get around reasonably well. Their brains learn to adapt and pay more attention to any balance system information that is still reliable.

But, as you now realize, people with damaged vestibular systems are not as steady on their feet as they once were. In fact, if the damage is severe in both ears, they may lurch and stagger–much like the proverbial "drunken sailor." Such people often use canes or walking sticks to help steady themselves. Even so, I don't know of any that are confined to wheelchairs solely because of their Ménière's. They are just running on the four smaller cylinders now.

If you have damaged both vestibular systems, you will have a much more difficult time when it is dark (when you can't use your eyes effectively) (you lose your two middle-sized cylinders) or when walking on uneven or soft ground (which messes up your proprioceptive system) (and thus you lose your two small cylinders). Under such conditions you will essentially have no balance and will have to "hang on" to a wall or another person.

By now you should have developed a sense of awe at the marvelous balance system God designed for you.[2] At the same time, you now realize the tremendous upsets that may come into your life and lifestyle as Ménière's disease damages this wonderful system.

Chapter 2 Endnotes

1 Bauman, 2011.
2 Bauman, 2011.

Chapter 3

How Do Doctors Diagnose Ménière's Disease?

Since Ménière's disease isn't a disease as such, but rather, a collection of symptoms, there are no definitive diagnostic tests to prove you have Ménière's disease. Furthermore, there are many disorders that present the same or similar symptoms as Ménière's disease. This makes diagnosing Ménière's disease most difficult.

Doctors typically diagnose the presence of Ménière's disease both by the presence of its four symptoms—fluctuating hearing loss, tinnitus, periodic episodes of vertigo and a feeling of fullness in the affected ear—and on the basis of differential diagnosis—ruling out all other conditions with somewhat similar symptoms.

In practical terms, Ménière's disease is the default diagnosis when your doctor has ruled out all the other possibilities through differential diagnosis. Thus, if he can't find any other condition, he concludes that you must have Ménière's disease.

To help him with his diagnosis, your doctor may subject you to a battery of tests as he tries to rule out one condition or another. Some of these tests include:

- **Audiogram:** to determine the kind (conductive, sensorineural) and degree of hearing loss by frequency.

- **Auditory brainstem response (ABR) testing:** sometimes called Brainstem Auditory Evoked Response (BAER), to track sound signals to, and in, your brain.
- **Balance testing:** including such tests as electronystagmography (ENG), rotational chair test, platform posturography, etc. These tests show your degree of balance function in each ear.
- **Blood testing:** to rule out conditions such as syphilis.
- **Computerized tomography (CT) scans of your head:** to rule out abnormalities in your ears and brain.
- **Electrocochleography (ECOG):** (a variant of the ABR test) to record thc electrical activity of the inner ear. It is used to rule out endolymphatic hydrops and perilymphatic fistulas.
- **Magnetic resonance imaging (MRI) of your head:** to rule out tumors in your brain or on your auditory nerves (acoustic neuromas).
- **Tympanometry:** to rule out Eustachian tube dysfunction.

The above tests help your doctor decide whether you have, or don't have, one or more of the conditions that are similar to, or mimic, Ménière's disease. Some of these similar conditions include:

- Acoustic neuromas. (Benign tumors on the acoustic nerve.)
- Autoimmune inner ear disease (AIED).
- Congenital ear malformations of various kinds.
- Impending strokes in the distribution of the anterior inferior cerebellar artery.
- Perilymph fistulas. (A tear in an inner ear membrane allowing perilymph to leak out.)
- Labyrinthitis, Vestibular neuritis (Often caused by a virus infecting the inner ear resulting in dizziness and vertigo if only vestibular neuritis, or, in addition, tinnitus and hearing loss if labyrinthitis. Onset of symptoms is usually abrupt, or you may wake up with them.)

- Lermoyez syndrome.
- Lyme disease.
- Migraines.
- Multiple sclerosis.
- Posterior fossa arachnoid cysts.
- Superior canal dehiscence syndrome (Tullio's Phenomenon).
- Syphilis.[1]

Lermoyez syndrome

At first glance, Lermoyez syndrome appears somewhat similar to Ménière's disease. Lermoyez syndrome consists of tinnitus and increasing hearing loss until an attack of dizziness (vertigo) occurs, after which, hearing rapidly improves.[2]

While Ménière's disease is chronic and progressive, Lermoyez syndrome is an acute phenomenon that results in no damage to the hair cells in the cochlea.[3]

In addition to these conditions, there are a number of other, rarer conditions that can also mimic Ménière's disease.

Complicating matters even more is the fact that people do not always get all the symptoms of classic Ménière's disease. Such people have atypical Ménière's disease. There are two versions of atypical Ménière's disease—cochlear hydrops and vestibular hydrops.

Cochlear hydrops is where you have excessive fluid in your cochlea. Vestibular hydrops is where you have excessive fluid in your semicircular canals. If you just have cochlear hydrops, you will not experience the vertigo or dizziness. However, you will still have the hearing loss, pressure in your ear and/or tinnitus. If you have vestibular hydrops, you will have the vertigo, pressure in your ear and/or tinnitus, but not the hearing loss.[4]

Doctors also sometimes refer to Ménière's disease as endolymphatic hydrops.[5] Almost, but not all people with Ménière's have endolymphatic hydrops. However, not all people with endolymphatic hydrops have Ménière's disease.[6]

Chapter 3 Endnotes

1 Hain, 2011a. p. 4.
2 Lermoyez syndrome, 2011. p. 1.
3 Wikipedia, 2011. p. 1.
4 Hines, 1997. p 3.
5 Rezen, 1985. p. 21.
6 Endolymphatic Hydrops, 1996. p. 2.

Chapter 4

What Causes Ménière's Disease?

The Historical Medical View

The exact cause of Ménière's disease has baffled doctors for the past 155 years. Although they have done much research over the years on Ménière's disease, medical researchers still don't know exactly what causes it.

In the past, researchers believed that the underlying cause of Ménière's disease was excess endolymph in certain chambers in your inner ears. They thought that the build-up of this excess endolymphatic fluid caused increased pressure, which, in turn, swelled the chambers containing the endolymph, thus damaging the delicate structures there. This resulted in the symptoms we call Ménière's disease.

Endolymphatic Hydrops

Doctors call this condition of excess fluid/pressure in your inner ears by the fancy name of "endolymphatic hydrops". ("Hydrops" is a medical term that means "excess fluid".)

Researchers also thought that endolymphatic hydrops was the result of either the body producing too much endolymph, or not draining it away fast enough through the endolymphatic duct and sac.

New research is changing this view. Researchers have now come to believe it is not so much the excess fluid itself, but the **fluctuating pressure** of the endolymph in the inner ear that causes the symptoms of Ménière's disease. Furthermore, they are leaning towards the opinion that this excess fluid is just a **marker** of Ménière's disease, rather than being responsible for the Ménière's symptoms.[1] Here's why.

First, contrary to most information written about Ménière's disease, hydrops is not found in all people with Ménière's disease. Furthermore, hydrops was also found in 6% of people who had no Ménière's symptoms, according to autopsy studies. In addition, although Ménière's disease occurs in approximately 2 out of every 1,000 people, hydrops is found in 60 out of every 1,000 people—30 **times** as many as you would expect if Ménière's disease was the result of hydrops.[2] Thus, logically, there must be other factors rather than simply hydrops involved in the origin of Ménière's disease.

> **Associated Conditions**
>
> Researchers "examined data from 1,376 self-reported Ménière's patients and 500,000 patients without Ménière's to look for correlations in who was more likely to experience this condition. They found that Ménière's disease was more prevalent in the elderly, in women, in Caucasians, and in patients with high body-mass indices. They also discovered that Ménière's patients were more likely to report co-morbid conditions related to allergies, immune dysfunction, autonomic dysfunction and poor mental health."[3]

Current medical thinking is that Ménière's disease is somehow related to immune system dysfunction diseases such as autoimmune inner ear disease (AIED). Autoimmune diseases may contribute a substantial percentage of the cases of Ménière's disease. For example, in one study about 25% of the people with Ménière's disease also had autoimmune thyroid disease.[4] There is evidence that genetics plays a role in immune system conditions and as such, AIED may be associated with Ménière's disease. In fact, more cases of Ménière's disease may be caused by immune system dysfunction than is presently thought.[5]

Taking this one step further, Dr. Mark Hyman has found that a lack of the body's powerful natural antioxidant glutathione can cause immune system dysfunction. One reason people may lack glutathione is they lack the GSTM1 gene, one of the key genes the body needs in order to make and recycle glutathione.[6] Thus, the basic underlying cause of Ménière's disease in some people could be genetic.

Here's how it would come about. Because the person lacks the GSTM1 gene, his body can't make/utilize enough glutathione to properly protect his immune system. As a result his immune system gets out of balance. This imbalance results in immune system dysfunction such as autoimmune problems. The autoimmune problems then show up in the form of Ménière's disease.

It may be that many/most cases of **bilateral** Ménière's disease are indeed related to immune system causes, and/or allergies. Dr. Hain reports that "about 16% of persons with bilateral Ménière's disease, and 6% of persons with Ménière's disease of any variety, may be due to immune dysfunction."[7]

Another interesting fact is that about 50% of the people with Ménière's disease get migraine headaches. Thus, it may be that migraines cause or trigger Ménière's disease in numbers of people.[8]

Today, medical doctors may attribute Ménière's symptoms to such things as auto-immune reactions, allergies, autonomic imbalances, blocked or damaged endolymphatic structures (This includes a smaller than normal endolymphatic sac that is not functioning properly. Thus, Ménière's disease may be viewed as a congenital disorder of the endolymphatic sac, and in this sense is probably hereditary.), viral infections of the inner ear, head injuries, vascular irregularities, metabolic disorders, damage to the ears from any cause that disturbs the balance of endolymph[9] and hereditary predispositions.[10,11]

As you can see from the above, doctors still do not clearly understand the underlying cause of Ménière's disease. However, researchers keep coming back to the idea that Ménière's disease is somehow associated with the build-up of excessive endolymphatic fluid in the balance (vestibular) portion of the inner ear. Autopsies on the bodies of people who were known to have had Ménière's disease have shown a ballooning of these chambers. This pretty much confirms the theory that high fluid pressure is involved in some way.

Dr. Hain explains,

> The fluid-filled hearing and balance structures of the inner ear normally function independently of the body's overall fluid/blood system. In a normal inner ear, the fluid is maintained at a constant volume and contains specific concentrations of sodium, potassium, chloride and other electrolytes. This fluid bathes the sensory cells of the inner ear and allows them to function normally.
>
> With injury or degeneration of the inner ear structures, independent control is lost, and the volume and concentration of the inner ear fluids fluctuate with changes in the body's fluid/blood. This fluctuation causes the symptoms of hydrops.[12]

Doctors still have not found out exactly why this happens. However, they believe that stress, excessive salt intake, endocrine problems, abnormal glucose (sugar) metabolism (diabetes), or an inability to handle fats are contributing factors.[13]

Endolymphatic Sac—the Body's Sodium Regulator?

Researchers have discovered "that the endolymphatic sac contains a substance that stimulates the kidneys to get rid of water and sodium. Although the nature of this substance, and how it is regulated, are yet unknown, it is tempting to speculate that the endolymphatic sac is involved in the body's system to regulate sodium concentration. If this proves to be true, it would explain why a low-sodium diet helps some people with Ménière's disease."[14]

In order to understand what happens in a Ménière's attack, you need to learn a little about the make-up of the inner ear. Your inner ears are bathed in two different fluids. The endolymph (the innermost fluid) is confined by membranes to the innermost parts of your inner ears (Fig. 4-1). Surrounding these membranes in your cochlea and vestibular (balance) parts of your inner ears is the perilymph. You could think of it as a balloon filled with endolymph suspended in a bowl of perilymph. The easy way to remember this is that endolymph is the inside (endo) fluid and the perilymph is "around the endolymph" (peri from which we get our English word "peripheral") fluid.

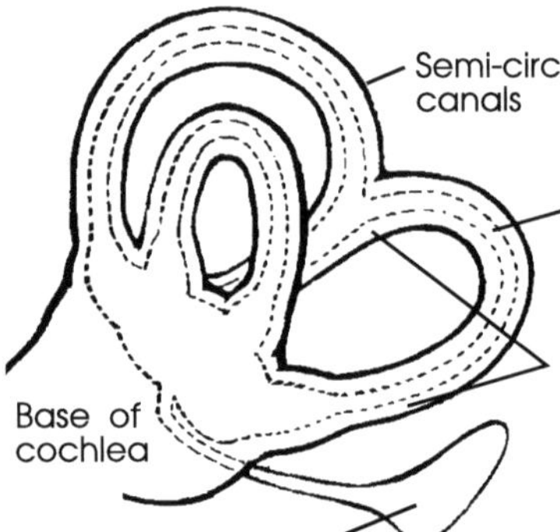

Fig. 4-1. The vestibular or balance system of your inner ears showing the three semi-circular canals. Endolymph fills the innermost parts of both your cochlea and your semi-circular canals. Surrounding this, and separated by a thin membrane, is the perilymph.

Both of these fluids contain electrolytes—substances that conduct electrical charges. Endolymph is rich in potassium and low in sodium. Perilymph is the opposite—rich in sodium and low in potassium. This sets up an electrical field. When a wave of sound stimulates the inner ear hair cells, they release chemicals that alter this electrical field. This excites the appropriate nerve cells. We perceive this as sound.[15]

In Ménière's disease, researchers believe your body produces too much endolymph, which builds up pressure. Perhaps this is what really happens. Your body constantly produces and absorbs endolymph. When something happens to slow down or stop this absorption process, excess fluid pressure results. This slowly increasing pressure irritates the inner ear. The result is increased tinnitus. At the same time, this excess pressure disturbs the basilar membrane, which contains the sound-sensing cells in the cochlea and causes a low-toned nerve-type (sensorineural) hearing loss.[16]

Normally the perilymph and the endolymph don't mix. Endolymph is a unique fluid. It uses potassium instead of sodium to generate ions. This results in a positive voltage of 85 mV between it and the surrounding perilymph.[18] When too much endolymph accumulates in the inner ear, the excess pressure ruptures the delicate membrane containing this fluid. The endolymph then spills out and mixes with the perilymph.

Endolymph—Just How Much Is Too Much?

Your ears contain extremely small amounts of endolymph. In each of your cochleae, for example, you have less than 2 ml (that's micro-liters—or 2 millionths of a liter) of endolymph.[17] That's about the volume of a piece of standard 0.5 mm mechanical pencil lead just over an inch long—very little indeed. Thus when we talk about "fluid build-up" we are really talking about minute amounts.

When these two different fluids mix, the combination essentially short-circuits the system.[19] The resulting hearing loss comes largely from injury to the sensory cells in the inner ear.[20]

Since the perilymph in your cochlea is connected to the perilymph in your vestibular system, you get instant dizziness (vertigo) or even "drop attacks". This is because the high potassium concentration in endolymph is toxic to the cells bathed by the perilymph causing them to swell and quit working properly—hence the instant vertigo.[21] Once the membranes heal and the fluid balance normalizes, the vertigo passes.[22]

The Current Upper Cervical View

As we have just seen, the medical view of Ménière's disease is wrapped up in a number of theories of what might cause Ménière's attacks in a few people. However, medical researchers still have not identified the basic underlying cause that results in these various symptoms in the vast majority of people with Ménière's. At best, they think these various symptoms are just markers of Ménière's—not the underlying cause. In short, medical researchers still don't have a clue as to the **underlying** cause of Ménière's disease. That's the bad news.

Dr. Burcon's Discovery

Now for some good news. Although medical doctors and medical science may not know much about the fundamental cause of Ménière's disease, and apparently have mostly been "barking up the wrong tree" all these years, that's not to say that no one knows anything about the basic causes of, and effective treatment for, Ménière's disease.

Surprisingly, one of the most common factors that results in Ménière's disease is quite simple to ascertain. Even better, the treatment can be fast, simple and painless. What's amazing is that it has taken all these years for someone to figure this out. Furthermore, the solution was serendipitous. It did not come about through dedicated scientific research. Here's the story.

In 1999, upper cervical chiropractor Dr. Michael Burcon made an intriguing finding. Three of his patients, who just happened to have Ménière's disease, quickly recovered from their vertigo after receiving upper-cervical-specific chiropractic treatments. Imagine the unmitigated joy these three patients experienced when they realized their vertigo, which had plagued them for years, had miraculously vanished. This is a far cry from how people with Ménière's sometimes come to him. As Dr. Burcon ruefully admits, "I've had people crawl down my office floor to the wastebasket and throw up from the nausea of Ménière's".[23]

One early patient explained,

> I suffered from Ménière's syndrome, or loss of balance, spinning and dizziness for **forty-five years**! I had all the things that went along with it: nausea, ringing in my ears, falling with the resulting broken bones and pain. It's a force that could really throw me to the floor at times. I could not look up or down, or lie flat, without the spinning starting immediately. So, to avoid falling, I learned to walk around by walls, and to keep my head steady or level and to hang onto everything. Michigan University Hospital in Ann Arbor, Wesley Memorial Hospital in Chicago and many neurosurgeons in Michigan, Illinois and Florida could do nothing to help me—only medication, which would make me sleep.
>
> Three months ago, Dr Michael Burcon gave me an [upper cervical chiropractic] treatment. I couldn't believe it. I was no longer dizzy! The next day, I realized all the ringing in my ears and other noises in my head were gone! I am still free from the dizzy spinning today. [24]

This and similar success stories from other patients got Dr. Burcon thinking. He began carefully documenting any cases of people with Ménière's disease that came to him. He soon realized that there was one thing in common that all the people with Ménière's disease that came to him had—and that was evidence of neck trauma—specifically, whiplash. Once he understood the cause, his chiropractic training suggested the treatment needed to correct this horrible condition. To date he has **successfully** treated more than 530 **consecutive** cases of people with Ménière's disease. That is not just an impressive success rate, it's a phenomenal success story, and one you need to know about if you have Ménière's disease and nothing else has worked for you.

The Physiology Underlying Ménière's Disease

There are a number of physical factors that seem to underlie Ménière's disease that medical doctors have missed. Here are some prominent ones.

The Atlas-Axis Connection

You have seven vertebrae in your neck numbered from C_1 through C_7. Your head sits directly on the C_1 vertebra, often called the "atlas" because it has a difficult job. (It got its name from Greek mythology where Atlas had the weight of the "celestial spheres" on his shoulders, just like your atlas vertebra has the weight of your head on it.)

Specifically, your head, which typically weighs around 10 or 11 pounds, rests on top of the two-ounce, doughnut-shaped atlas vertebra. The atlas is also called the "yes" bone because your head rocks back and forth on its two articulations when you nod your head to indicate "yes". That is why, when your skull slips partially off one of these atlas joints in one direction or another, pressure is applied to the brain stem, causing you to be "off your rocker"![25] As Dr. Burcon explains, "Ménière's is a nasty disease, but we can usually help people get their heads on straight".[26]

Your second vertebra (C_2) is called the "axis". This is the vertebra that allows you to turn your head left and right. You could call it the "no" bone because it allows your head to rotate left and right as you shake your head "no".

Incidentally, your atlas and axis are the only two vertebrae that do not have inter-vertebral discs between them like the rest of the vertebrae in your spine have. Furthermore, they are the two most freely moveable vertebrae, and as a result, are the ones most commonly misaligned and the easiest to be misaligned.[27]

You might not realize this, but your brainstem actually extends down into the atlas and axis cavity so your spinal cord basically begins with the C_3 vertebra. Thus, if your top two vertebrae are out of alignment (what chiropractors call a subluxation), they put pressure on the base of your brainstem. This, in turn, interferes with the free flow of signals up and down your nervous system—sometimes with serious consequences. As Dr. Burcon explains, "Five of the twelve cranial nerves originate in the brainstem. The base of the brain controls many important bodily functions, such as breathing, blood pressure, the sleep center, and balance."

When a C_1 or C_2 subluxation occurs, the weight of your head is no longer balanced evenly on your atlas. Rather, it is moved off center because of head tilt. When this happens, the rest of your body will begin to compensate for that shift of weight. One shoulder will drop down, one hip will come up bringing a leg up with it creating imbalance in your body. Now you have a problem with your back. One leg appears relatively shorter than the other and you are not walking with a normal gait.[28]

As we have just seen, this head-neck misalignment results in pressure on the brainstem. This can cause interference at the point where your head and neck join (the atlas). "If the atlas is out of its proper position, it can irritate, constrict or disrupt vital nerve signals to any portion of your body. This can cause muscle or joint pain, organ dysfunction, lowered immune system and countless other conditions that you would not ordinarily relate to a problem originating in your neck"[29] including the symptoms of Ménière's disease. Therefore, in order to maintain good health, it is important for you to keep your head "screwed on straight".

From the side, you want your spine to have a nice curve to it. If the atlas is subluxated, it takes the curve out of your spine. However, as seen from the front or back you want your spine to be straight, not curved sideways in any place.[30]

This is where upper cervical chiropractic treatment comes in. Adjusting the atlas (and axis) can take this pressure off your brainstem, thus alleviating many problems by allowing your brain to send its healing messages throughout your body and allowing your spine to revert to its proper alignment.

The Endolymph Connection

As we saw in Chapter 3, Ménière's disease is also called "endolymphatic hydrops". Endolymphatic hydrops, according to the Merck Manual, is defined as, "The accumulation of the fluid of the membranous labyrinth of the ear, thought to be caused by the over production or under absorption of that fluid".

Earlier in this chapter, we explained that your inner ear consists of two fluids, endolymph and perilymph. When everything is working correctly, your body continually produces new endolymph, and at the same time—since your inner ear is a closed system—absorbs an equal amount of the existing endolymph, thus maintaining a constant endolymphatic pressure.

Also, as we saw earlier in this chapter, medical doctors keep coming back to the idea that Ménière's disease is somehow associated with the build-up of excessive endolymph (endolymphatic fluid) in the balance (vestibular) portion of the inner ear. This only happens if something upsets this delicate system so that your body produces too much endolymph or cannot absorb the existing endolymph fast enough. When something impairs your body's ability to properly regulate the amount of endolymph in your inner ears, such as pressure on your vestibulo-cochlear nerve from a subluxation of the atlas, you can end up with Ménière's disease. Thus the real problem underlying Ménière's disease isn't found in your inner ear, but is caused by having your atlas/axis vertebrae out of proper alignment.

The Whiplash Connection

Whiplash can knock you "off your rocker". Dr. Burcon has positively established a link between both Ménière's disease and trigeminal neuralgia with whiplash injuries that misalign the base of your skull with the top of your neck. This creates a lesion affecting your Eustachian tubes and/or the trigeminal ganglion. Whiplash injuries set the stage, and then other conditions may eventually follow.

For example, you may also get bad facial pain (trigeminal neuralgia) because of head/neck trauma or whiplash injuries when you were quite young. Your first indication may be Bell's palsy. It may go away spontaneously and then a worse condition comes along.[31]

One thing Dr. Burcon has found in his research of 530 consecutive Ménière's patients is that they all have one thing in common. Their X-rays show that they have significant whiplash injury from falling on their heads or from car accidents. According to Dr. Burcon, about half of these traumas were caused by vehicle accidents and the other half from injuries involving head trauma. Interestingly enough, most of his patients deny these earlier injuries because they happened so long ago that they have forgotten about them, or they didn't take them seriously in the first place.[32]

In addition, Greg Buchanan, who suffered for years as a result of an atlas/axis subluxation, further explains,

> Simple accidents such as falling from a bike and hitting your head, hitting your head on a door jam or bedside table, sustaining a head, neck or shoulder injury when playing contact sports can, and do, result in these subluxations.[33]

In layman's terms, basically whiplash is when the vertebrae in your neck are "out" such that your head gets stuck tipped forward and off to one side. This irritates the nerves in your autonomic nervous system so they don't work properly. In addition, blood flow is reduced in the cervical area. So is the flow of cerebral-spinal fluid (CFS) to the inner ear. This is important since, as we previously noted, Ménière's disease is thought to be related to problems with excess endolymph in your inner ear. Furthermore, when the 5th cranial nerve (trigeminal nerve) is compressed, it affects your soft palate so it quits working right, thus affecting proper Eustachian tube function. In turn, this causes the feelings of fullness in your middle ear on the side affected by Ménière's disease. The 5th cranial nerve also controls the proper functioning of your temporo-mandibular joint (TMJ) which also can affect Eustachian tube function. Finally, when the 8th cranial nerve (the vestibulo-cochlear nerve) is affected, it can result in low-frequency hearing loss, tinnitus and balance conditions such as vertigo and dizziness.[34] Who would have guessed that a single neck bone could cause all these problems and result in what we call Ménière's disease?

The Subluxation Connection

Chiropractors talk about subluxations. In medical terms a "luxation" is a complete dislocation of two bones. Thus, a subluxation is an incomplete luxation (slight dislocation). A subluxation occurs when the alignment between two bones is altered, yet at the same time, the two joint surfaces remain in contact with each other (Stedman's Medical Dictionary).

Subluxations may be quite small—only 1 or 2 mm—but this is enough to cause problems. Medical doctors typically discount these slight subluxations as not being medically significant. Typically, when they read cervical X-rays, they say everything is normal because they can't see any broken bones, or they can't see any tumors. Furthermore, they think any misalignments will right themselves on their own. However, the truth is that if you get a reverse curve in your neck, the only way to get that curve restored to normal is if you go to an skilled chiropractor according to Dr. Burcon.[35]

In addition, if you get a vertebra out in your neck, you will usually end up with lower back pain because, as Dr. Burcon says,

> Your spine starts adapting and compensating and twisting trying to take the pressure off your brainstem, and the vertebrae will move in several directions to keep you upright.

This is because,

> If your body has to choose between your head and your lower back, it will sacrifice your lower back in order to keep your eyes and ears level so you don't get dizzy.[36]

"Misalignments in other spinal vertebrae", according to Dr. Blair, the father of the Blair method of upper cervical spine chiropractic, "require far more force to occur and are usually as a result of significant trauma. They are usually secondary to an upper cervical subluxation."[37]

Greg Buchanan adds,

> I find a high correlation between many diseases or medical conditions and one particular condition or state. In medical literature it is known as an occipitio-atlantal (C_0 to C_1) [head to atlas] subluxation and can be accompanied by an atlanto-axial (C_1 to C_2) [atlas to axis] subluxation.[38]

There are basically 4 directions an atlas subluxation can occur according to the Blair method of chiropractic treatment. It can either be:

1. Anterior (in front of) and Superior (above) on the Right
2. Anterior (in front of) and Superior (above) on the Left
3. Posterior (behind) and Inferior (below) on the Right
4. Posterior (behind) and Inferior (below) on the Left.[39]

A head injury may result in the skull/atlas shifting to one of these four positions. Such movement is dependent upon the amplitude of the force, the direction it comes from and the anatomy of the person sustaining the force. A consequence of the injury can be ligaments stretching and/or tearing. This can result in the person's head remaining in a subluxated position and requiring intervention of some kind to restore the normal skull/atlas relationship and head and neck realignment.[40]

Note that an atlas subluxation both posterior (behind) and inferior (below) on the right (No. 3 above) can irritate the 8th cranial nerve (the vestibulo-cochlear nerve that controls balance and hearing) on the left side and that can lead to the symptoms of Ménière's disease.[41]

It is interesting that Ménière's disease generally occurs in only one ear at a time. Furthermore, which ear it occurs in is determined to a large extent by the direction of the subluxation. The following table is based on the results Dr. Burcon obtained from examining 300 Ménière's patients.

No. of occurrences	Direction of Subluxation and Ear Involved
0	Anterior (in front of) and Superior (above) on the opposite side to the involved ear
18	Anterior (in front of) and Superior (above) on the same side as the involved ear
12	Posterior (behind) and Inferior (below) on the same side as the involved ear
270	Posterior (behind) and Inferior (below) on the opposite side to the involved ear[42]

Notice that in 90% of the cases, the atlas subluxation is behind and below on the **opposite** side to the ear with Ménière's disease. Thus, this is the condition the overwhelming majority of people with Ménière's disease have. However, if you have been in multiple accidents, or in an accident that caused more than one blow to your head, the subluxations can be in opposite (or any) directions.[43]

In an earlier study of just the first 30 Ménière's patients Dr. Burcon treated, he discovered that prior to the onset of their symptoms, all 30 people suffered cervical traumas; most from automobile accidents, resulting in previously-undiagnosed whiplash injuries. These patients all had the same subluxation that resulted in Ménière's disease as the 270 cases (above). At that time, Dr. Burcon noted,

> It cannot be coincidental that thirty consecutive Ménière's patients would present with a posterior and inferior atlas listing with laterality on the opposite side of the involved ear.[44]

Note: Many more people suffer whiplash and other cervical trauma than have Ménière's disease. One reason everyone doesn't end up with Ménière's disease from an atlas/axis subluxation is because they didn't get the specific subluxation that Dr. Burcon has found to result in Ménière's disease (bottom line in the above table). Other subluxations don't seem to cause Ménière's disease (or at least not very often), but they can certainly cause a number of other problems in your body. (See the next section.) Therefore, it is a good idea to have your atlas/axis checked by a upper cervical chiropractor after any occurrences of whiplash or other head/neck trauma if you desire to remain in good health.

Incidentally, the C_1 and C_2 vertebrae are intimately related. As a result, if one goes out, the other is also probably out too. They both usually move in the same direction.[45] However, they are not necessarily "out" by the same amount.

Dr. Burcon further explains,

> When the **atlas** is the **major** subluxation, vertigo with vomiting is the major symptom. However, when the **axis** is the **major** subluxation, hearing loss, ear fullness and tinnitus are the major symptoms.[46]

This is why if only one vertebra is "off", you may have incomplete Ménière's disease—what doctors sometimes call vestibular hydrops (in the case of an atlas subluxation) and cochlear hydrops (in the case of an axis subluxation).

Also, it often happens that subluxations occur in pairs. The most common subluxation pair are the atlas and C_5 vertebrae. The next most common pair are the axis and C_6 vertebrae. The third most common pair are the atlas and axis together. People with both their atlas and axis "out" typically cannot drive or work. They rarely leave their homes.[47]

If your C_5 vertebra is "out" as well as your atlas (C_1), you may experience a number of problems with your body in addition to your major Ménière's symptoms of vertigo and associated vomiting. As Dr. Burcon explains,

> When the C_5 vertebra is out, it messes up the vagus nerve and you could thus have digestion problems, or irritable bowel syndrome, or headaches, or pain in your arm, or tingling in your arm and hand. You could have pain in the joints in your arm. It could cause some problems with your lungs and breathing. It can contribute to panic attacks, also anxiety and depression as well.[48]

Not only do subluxations affect your nerves, they can also affect the blood supply to your inner ears (and other parts of your body). That is why right after an upper cervical treatment you may feel a rush of blood in your head. Some people's faces turn beet red for a bit as a result. The good news is that if the lack of an adequate supply of blood (and oxygen) to your inner ears has caused much of your hearing loss, you may experience a dramatic return of much of your hearing as your inner ears start working properly again. (This cannot happen if the hair cells are dead, but it does happen if the hair cells and other inner ear structures are just "sick" from lack of oxygen.)

The Multi-Symptom Connection

Because the atlas and axis vertebrae are the gateway to the rest of your body, when either or both of these vertebrae are "off", it prevents the nerves from working properly and transmitting healing messages to the rest of your body. The result is that a number of what seem to be unrelated problems can develop.

For example, about 50% of the people with Ménière's disease get migraine headaches. As you can see from the list below, migraine headaches can be caused by an atlas subluxation, so this makes sense.

In addition to causing Ménière's disease symptoms such as vertigo, dizziness, tinnitus, hearing loss and feelings of fullness in the ear, subluxations of the atlas and/or axis can cause a whole host of apparently-unrelated conditions such as, but not limited to:

- allergies, arthritis, asthma, arm pain, athletic injuries, attention deficit disorder
- back pain, bed wetting, Bell's palsy
- carpal tunnel syndrome, cerebral palsy, chronic fatigue, chronic infections, constipation
- depression, digestive problems
- epileptic seizures, ear infections, eye infections
- female disorders, fever, flu symptoms, frequent colds
- hacking cough, hay fever, headaches (all types), high (and low) blood pressure, hip pain
- immune system deficiency, indigestion, infertility
- knee pain
- leg pain, loss of sleep, low back pain
- migraine headaches, muscle spasms
- neck pain, nervousness, neuralgia, neuritis, numbness
- pain (chronic), poor vision
- restlessness
- shoulder pain, sinus problems, sore throat
- tendonitis, tight muscles, tingling sensations, temporomandibular dysfunction (TMD), trigeminal neuralgia
- whiplash.[49]

Obviously, all the above conditions can have more than one cause, but as Dr. Burcon says, "I always keep going back and back in a person's case history and I start to see these progressions over time—one thing after another that are seemingly unrelated,"[50] yet most of these conditions are the ultimate result of the upper cervical spine being out of alignment.

For example, one of the major causes of back pain is having your neck out of place for a long time. Since it takes a long time before you begin to have the back pain, when you finally go to your doctor about your lower back pain, he doesn't ask you about your neck, so neck trauma from "way back" gets overlooked as the primary cause.[51]

The good news is that by adjusting the atlas and axis (and any other vertebrae) that need adjusting, upper cervical chiropractors can generally alleviate, and often eliminate, the above conditions.

The Time Connection

One of the interesting things about Ménière's disease resulting from whiplash and other head trauma is that typically there is an average delay of 15 years between the time of the head trauma and the appearance of the Ménière's disease symptoms.[52]

Probably this long latency period is why no one previously saw the correlation between whiplash and Ménière's disease until Dr. Burcon came along. (This also applies to trigeminal neuralgia.)

This is also probably why few people are diagnosed with Ménière's disease at a younger age. Remember, this 15-year delay is the **average** delay. Some people have their Ménière's symptoms appear much sooner (and obviously this is what happens when children and young adults get Ménière's disease), and some have a greater delay than 15 years.

In any event, people typically are diagnosed with Ménière's disease in middle age—around age 40 or so—yet their injuries most often happened 15 to 25 years previously during their high school or college years. For example, they may have been in a car accident when they were learning to drive or soon after—during their reckless driving years. They may have had one or more sports injuries in high school or college. They may have done some dumb stunts in their youth or in college that resulted in "falling on their heads".

Furthermore, few people list these old injuries on their doctor's admission paperwork. In fact, they have often long-since forgotten about them. Thus, they fail to make any connection with these old injuries and their current Ménière's disease symptoms.

The Genetic Connection

Some people feel that Ménière's disease runs in families, and thus there must be a genetic connection. In truth, Ménière's disease may have something to do with genetics. You see, Ménière's disease can run in families because family members likely have similar bone structures, and some varieties of these bone structures may be more susceptible to misalignment.[53]

For example, you may be big-boned or small boned. That is a genetic trait you inherited from your parents. You may wonder what this has to do with Ménière's disease. If you have big bones, you will have larger vertebrae and larger holes in the center for the spinal nerves to pass through. If you have smaller bones, your vertebrae likely will have smaller holes in their centers.

You may also have larger or smaller nerves (another genetic trait). If you have large bones and small nerves, obviously your atlas could have a subluxation to some degree and still not "pinch" your nerves. In contrast, if you have small bones and larger nerves, even just a tiny subluxation could put pressure your nerves and lower brainstem and result in things such as Ménière's disease.

As chiropractor Dr. Robert Brooks explains,

> Some people have big bones and little nerves. Thus, most of their problems are going to be structural. Some people have bigger nerves and smaller bones and they are going to have all kinds of neurological and functional complications with that structure. Furthermore, some people have a combination of both and their problems will go in both directions.

This is just one example of how genetics can play a role in whether you experience Ménière's disease or not.

Putting It All Together

As we have seen, Ménière's disease symptoms almost always initially stem from whiplash or similar head trauma. In addition, there may be a number of other factors that together result in an upper cervical subluxation complex.[54]

They call it a complex for a good reason. Not only have you had an upper cervical misalignment for a long time, but there are a lot of different components. With Ménière's disease, as Dr. Burcon explains,

> You have different symptoms, different intensities, different cycles. You could have an autoimmune component. There could be less blood going to the inner ear. There could be too much pressure in the cerebrospinal fluid. (There are two main fluids inside the skull which is an enclosed hydraulic system. If the blood pressure is too low, the other pressure is too high.)[55]
>
> Furthermore, Ménière's disease involves the 8th cranial nerve (the vestibulo-cochlear nerve that controls both the hearing and balance systems). When this nerve is compressed, it can result in an inner-ear symptom complex consisting of attacks of vertigo, low-frequency hearing loss, and tinnitus.
>
> In addition, Ménière's disease is not just an inner ear problem. It is also a middle ear syndrome highlighted by Eustachian tube dysfunction (e.g. feeling of fullness) compounded by dysfunction of the temporomandibular joints.[56]
>
> This is because Ménière's disease also has to do with the trigeminal nerve. (The trigeminal or 5th cranial nerve is responsible for sensations and motor functions in the face and jaw.) Among other things, the trigeminal nerve opens and closes the muscle in the middle ear. When the trigeminal nerve is not working correctly, it can result in Eustachian tube dysfunction. This is often why people with Ménière's disease don't like big pressure changes from the weather. The other end of the Eustachian tube lies right between the C_1 and C_2 vertebrae so swelling there can close up the opening of the Eustachian tube. That's why sometimes when a plane is landing, the rapid pressure changes can set off a Ménière's attack. Even getting up too quickly can cause an attack.[57]
>
> In support of this view, note "that insertion of a middle-ear ventilation tube can temporarily alleviate Ménière's symptoms, suggesting Eustachian tube dysfunction (ETD) as a contributing factor. Furthermore, clinical practice also shows that treating disorders of the upper and lower cervical spine and temporomandibular joints can lessen Ménière's disease symptoms."[58]

Also, "stellate ganglion blocks [injecting a local anesthetic to temporarily numb the sympathetic nerves] can be beneficial in controlling Ménière's disease symptoms, highlighting the influence of the autonomic nervous system".[59] The stellate ganglion are a collection of sympathetic nerves located on each side of your voice box at the level of the sixth and seventh cervical vertebrae (the last vertebra in your neck).

Another factor is that you can have a systemic virus like the herpes virus, so you can have an infection in your ear, and that can contribute to some of these things including Eustachian tube dysfunction. It may be any kind of viral infection, or any other type of infection for that matter.[60]

As you can see, there are many factors that can be involved in Ménière's disease, but it always seems to come back to the underlying fact that the atlas and/or axis vertebrae are out of proper alignment.

In fact, Dr. Burcon has proved that Ménière's disease is primarily the result of the subluxation of the atlas and/or axis vertebrae. For example, he found that 470 consecutive patients, diagnosed with Ménière's by ENTs, and coming to his practice for care of vertigo, tested positive for upper cervical subluxations. He then took three cervical X-rays of each patient. Analysis of these X-rays confirmed the presence of such subluxations, and also showed evidence of whiplash—in spite of the fact that more than 50% of these patients denied that had had any cervical trauma.[61]

After treating these 470 consecutive people with Ménière's disease using upper cervical techniques, the results were impressive. "Long-term neurophysiological improvements after **initial** adjustments have been clinically documented in ninety percent of these cases."[62]

Reduction in **vertigo** for Ménière's patients is similarly impressive. Before treatment, on a scale of 0 to 10 with 0 being no vertigo and 10 being the worst vertigo imaginable, these 470 patients rated their vertigo (both frequency and intensity combined) at an average of about 7.8.

Six weeks after initial treatment they again rated their vertigo, but now their frequency/intensity rating dramatically fell to just 2.8 (a 64% reduction) That alone would make most Ménière's sufferers ecstatic! But that's not all.

At one year post treatment, vertigo frequency/intensity ratings dropped to about 1.8, and by the end of two years post treatment, these ratings were down to 1.2.

Even more impressive, by the end of 3 years these ratings dropped to less than 0.1! In other words, by the end of 3 years, you essentially do not have problems with vertigo anymore![63] That is wonderful news!

Chapter 4 Endnotes

1 Hain, 2011a. p. 2.
2 Hain, 2011a. p. 3.
3 Tyrrell, 2014. p. 28.

4 Hain, 2011a. p. 3.
5 Hain, 2010c. p. 2.
6 Hyman, 2010. p. 2.
7 Hain, 2010c, p. 1.
8 Hain, 2011a. p. 3.
9 Shea, 1993. pp. 224-229.
10 Salt, 1998b. p. 1.
11 Hain, 2011a. p. 3.
12 Hain, 2011a. p. 9.
13 Ménière's Disease, 1997. p. 2.
14 Ménière's Disease and the Meniett Low-Pressure Pulse Generator, 2002. p. 2.
15 Vernick, 1993. p. 16.
16 Salt, 1998f. p. 1.
17 Salt, 1998g. p. 1.
18 Salt, 1998e. p. 1.
19 Vernick, 1993. p. 16.
20 Vernick, 1993. pp. 172-173.
21 Salt, 1998f. p. 2.
22 Engel, 1993. p. 161.
23 Burcon, 2015a.
24 Heselsweet, 1999.
25 Burcon, 2015b.
26 Burcon, 2015a.
27 Buchanan, 2015a.
28 Burcon, 2015c.
29 Upper Cervical Chiropractic, 2015.
30 Burcon, 2015c.
31 Burcon, 2015c.
32 Burcon, 2015c.
33 Buchanan, 2015b.
34 Burcon, 2010.
35 Burcon, 2015c.
36 Burcon, 2015c.
37 Buchanan, 2015a.
38 Buchanan, 2015b.
39 Burcon, ~2011.
40 Burcon, 2015a.
41 Burcon, 2005.
42 Burcon, ~2011.
43 Burcon, 2015c.
44 Burcon, 2005.
45 Burcon, 2015c.
46 Burcon, ~2011.
47 Burcon, ~2011
48 Burcon, 2015c.
49 Buchanan, 2015c.
50 Burcon, 2015c.
51 Burcon, 2015c.
52 Burcon, 2010.
53 Burcon, 2015c.
54 Burcon, ~2011
55 Burcon, 2015c.

56 Burcon, ~2011.
57 Burcon, 2015c.
58 Burcon, ~2011.
59 Burcon, ~2011.
60 Burcon, 2015c.
61 Burcon, 2010.
62 Burcon, 2005.
63 Burcon, ~2011.

Chapter 5

Treatments for Ménière's Disease

Since the fundamental underlying cause of Ménière's disease relates to subluxations in the atlas and axis vertebrae, it stands to reason that the first thing you want to do if you are diagnosed with Ménière's disease is go to an upper cervical spine chiropractor and have him check out your C_1 and C_2 vertebrae (and indeed, your whole spine).

Upper Cervical Treatment

Now that you have learned just how valuable upper cervical chiropractic treatment can be in treating your Ménière's disease, you might ask, "Can't I just go to any chiropractor for upper cervical treatment? Aren't all chiropractors trained in spinal adjustments?"

The answer is "Yes". All chiropractors **are** trained in spinal adjustments, but their training does not prepare them to be **experts** in specifically adjusting the atlas and axis vertebrae!

Conventional chiropractors are people who have attended a recognized chiropractic school and received their Doctor of Chiropractic degree (DC). To obtain this degree they must first earn a 4-year bachelor level degree followed by a 4-year doctoral degree in chiropractic.

All upper cervical chiropractors have earned DC degrees, but they have also gone on to take a 1-year post-doctoral specialty in upper cervical spine treatment techniques and associated clinical training. Only about 2% of chiropractors go on to take the upper cervical post-doctoral training, but even so, there are upper cervical chiropractors scattered around the country.

Another question you might be asking is, "If upper cervical chiropractic is so wonderful, and works so well for Ménière's disease and other conditions, how come I've never heard of it before?"

There are two main reasons. First, the medical community typically has been, and largely still is, strongly prejudiced against chiropractic. Thus, medical doctors don't tell their Ménière's patients about upper cervical chiropractic and how it can help them. This keeps their patients in the dark about effective upper cervical treatments and thus keeps them coming back to their doctors again and again for treatment rather than letting them go elsewhere and be cured. (Can't you hear the money talking here?)

Second,

> There are laws in every state and Canada that prevent chiropractors that use any particular procedure, whether upper cervical or otherwise, from freely advertising the procedure they have dedicated their lives to learning. One law in particular forbids any chiropractor that uses any particular procedure to infer that his method is superior or more advanced than other chiropractic methods.[1]

There are a number of different approaches to upper cervical chiropractic adjustments—about 10 or so. All of them require extra training. Furthermore, all of them require extra time with each patient. Dr. Burcon is partial to the "hands-on" Blair method, but he is quick to point out that the other methods are all good too.

In addition to the Blair method for treating the upper cervical spine, some of other methods include the Atlas Orthogonal, the HIO (Hole-in-One) Toggle Recoil, the Kale Brainstem, the NUCCA, the Knee Chest, the Orthospinology/ Grostic, the Quantum Spinal Mechanics and the Palmer Specific to name some of the more common ones. You can learn more about these various upper cervical treatment methods at http://www.upcspine.com/tech.htm.

Each of these methods have their unique advantages in certain situations. As Dr. Burcon explains, "There is no one chiropractic technique that works best for every patient, every time."[2] For any given patient, one method may be better than the others for some reason.[3] Since everyone is made slightly differently, each person may need one or another of the various treatment methods.

Upper cervical treatments are for the most part gentle. Greg Buchanan explains,

> Upper cervical spine chiropractors utilize very specific, and mainly gentle approaches, techniques, methods and procedures to measure and

> "adjust" displacements [subluxations] in the upper cervical vertebrae—in particular, displacements of the atlas with respect to the skull. There are quite a few approaches, which differ in analysis, and adjustment technique, but overwhelmingly they are gentle, very accurate and very effective. Those people who have been ill, who have a confirmed subluxation of their atlas and who have received a professional and well-executed upper cervical adjustment to the atlas will testify to the adjustment's effectiveness. Just like me, they have seen the benefits of this wonderful alternative health approach.[4]

The Upper-Cervical website (http:www.upper-cervical.com) explains it this way.

> The upper cervical correction can be described as a slight predetermined direction of pressure applied to the first bone (atlas) or second bone (axis) in the neck. Depending on the technique, it can feel like a brisk thrust, a light tap, or a massage on the side of the neck just below the earlobe. That's where the atlas is. Sometimes this is accompanied by a loud pop or series of tiny ticks as the bone moves back into place.[5]

If you are worried about chiropractors being too rough and jerking you around and cracking you up, you'll be in for a pleasant surprise. You see, upper cervical chiropractors do not "manipulate" your neck; they "adjust" it. This adjustment technique is quite tolerable, non-invasive and involves no twisting or cracking of your neck.

Buchanan explains,

> Cutting through the noise about manipulation, it's important to understand that there is a **huge** difference between "manipulation" and "adjustment". True upper cervical spine chiropractors don't just grab your head and twist your neck "hoping" to unlock, some "locked" vertebrae. Nor do they crack, crunch, rotate, or take your neck to its full range of motion and move it with high velocity in the other direction. This type of approach is what I would call manipulation.
>
> Upper cervical spine chiropractors, on the other hand, are very deliberate and very measured in their approach. They measure displacements in upper cervical vertebrae with accuracy, utilizing precision X-rays to analyze such displacements thoroughly in order to determine the best direction of the adjusting force to achieve the best result possible. This specific before and after measurement and correction is the hallmark of the upper cervical spine chiropractor and determines the difference, in my opinion between manipulation and adjustment.[6]

When choosing an upper cervical chiropractor, you want to make sure that your chiropractor uses specific measuring techniques so he knows what is "out", and which way it is "out". After treatment, you want to be sure your chiropractor has ways of knowing that the atlas and axis are now in proper alignment.

One technique many chiropractors use is to have you lay on your stomach. They then compare your leg lengths. (Typically they check that the back of the heels on your shoes match exactly.) If any vertebrae are "out", typically your spine shifts, which tilts your pelvis, resulting in one leg appearing shorter than the other. They then adjust your spine so it is in proper alignment. When they do this, your pelvis returns to level, and thus both of your legs now appear the same length.

Unfortunately conventional chiropractors often treat your lower back to get your pelvis level again, but fail to properly treat the atlas and axis. As Dr. Burcon explains,

> The chiropractor that is hurrying pushes on the longest leg and straightens out your lower back and your legs are now balanced. However, 15 minutes later, it pops back out because the real problem originated from your neck. Furthermore, most conventional chiropractors don't let you rest for 15 minutes or so, then recheck your vertebrae to make sure the adjustments are holding.[7]

Apart from the leg-length check, Dr. Burcon feels that every chiropractor should have at least two totally different ways to check that he has adjusted things correctly—such as the X-ray and thermography methods he uses. He explains,

> I think that it is most important that you're good at a couple of different ways, otherwise you might miss something. There's no one test that works for everyone 100% of the time. You need two different checking systems, but that doesn't always have to be thermography. You could pick something else, practicing to learn how to do it well.[8]

He continues,

> I use X-rays. I always take X-rays before, but not always after, especially if a patient doesn't want many X-rays taken. As for post-treatment X-rays, sometimes the insurance company wants one, sometimes the patient wants one, sometimes I need one for my research, but I don't do a whole lot of post-treatment X-rays.
>
> If you are doing well, I probably wouldn't take another X-ray for a year if we were getting the results that we were looking for and I didn't need more information or confirmation.

> If you just go by feel (challenges) you will be right about 85% of the time, but that is not good enough for me. That is why I take X-rays. B. J. Palmer, who started the specific cervical treatments, said you couldn't be specific without an X-ray. He was one of the first chiropractors to buy an X-ray machine.
>
> The second method I use is thermography. Thermography is only measuring the heat you are giving off. Thus, there is no X-ray radiation to worry about. As a result, you can take as many thermographs as you want without any danger to the patient. Most Blair chiropractors use thermography as their second way to check their adjustments.
>
> With thermography, I take heat pictures of your neck. I can do your back too if you complain of problems in your back. Over time I've learned to see certain patterns. You can see which vertebra is lighting up and is too hot, and which leg is too short and how things change when you use different methods. You have to tailor your methods of treatment to each individual person because each person is different. Too many chiropractors use the same adjustments on everybody because they are going for quantity (more patients), not quality.[9]

After you have had an upper cervical chiropractic treatment you need to be very careful not to put your neck "out" again. Thus, an important part of the treatment is to lay down and rest for 20 minutes or so right there in the chiropractors office, after which, a good chiropractor will recheck your neck to be sure it is still in proper alignment.

Some good upper cervical chiropractors tell their patients who drive to their appointments to back their cars into a parking stall so they can drive out without turning their necks too far like they would have to if they were backing out of a parking spot.

Doing this helps you prevent your atlas and axis from going "out" again before you even get home. It takes time for your ligaments, tendons and muscles to shrink and hold the proper alignment again. Thus you may have to have several adjustments in short order to keep them in place while they heal.

Thus the question arises, "How often do I have to have an upper cervical chiropractic treatment?" The answer is that it depends on your own body. You see, your vertebrae may not stay in place after the initial treatment because, by the time you sought treatment, your ligaments, tendons and muscles had all been stretched out of shape for a number of years, and it takes time for them to shrink and get used to holding your vertebrae in their proper positions again. This is why initially "some people have to be corrected once or twice a week, or even more often, then one or twice a month. Other people can hold their correction for several months, even a year at a time. Everyone is different."

One rule of thumb is that it will take roughly one month for every year the subluxation existed. This means that if your vertebrae were "out" for 12 years, you could expect it could take up to 12 months for your body to completely adjust, and for your vertebrae learn to stay in their correct positions. Remember, this is just a rule of thumb. For some people their symptoms disappear soon after the first treatment. For others, it takes months. As Dr. Burcon explains, "Relief may be instantaneous but sometimes it has to run its course."

"The upper cervical doctor's objective is to make as precise an upper cervical correction as possible. Then, he must help you maintain the correction with as few corrections as possible so that you may live pain-free and enjoy a better quality of life."[10]

After upper cervical treatment, your Ménière's and other symptoms may decrease immediately, or pain may change and move to another area of your body. This is a good sign that your body is now busy healing itself.

Dr. Burcon's typical chiropractic treatment includes a detailed case history, including a letter from the patient's ENT and copies of all the ENT's tests used to diagnose Ménière's disease. He takes cervical thermographs (using a Titronics TyTron C-3000). He performs a modified Prill leg check analysis. He takes 3 modified Blair cervical X-rays. Then, after careful analysis of the above, he makes adjustments to the upper cervical spine based on his analysis. Finally, the patient lays down for a 15-minute rest after which Dr. Burcon rechecks him to be sure everything is still in alignment.[11]

Retracing May Take Time

Chiropractic adjustments may result in almost instantaneous healing, or they may take time to restore your body to a healthy condition again depending on how long you have had the condition. A good rule of thumb is that acute (recent) cases respond rapidly, while chronic (long-standing) conditions take more time. This is because with chronic conditions such as Ménière's disease, a number of years have passed from the time you were "healthy" until you reached your present condition with disabling Ménière's disease. Thus, you body needs time to heal itself.

When a chiropractor adjusts your vertebrae, the ligaments and muscles need time to regain their normal tone after having been stretched out of shape for years. Furthermore, your body often needs to rebuild some of these tissues in order for your vertebrae to hold their proper alignment. In addition, tissues that have assumed an abnormal condition over the years due to the gradually increasing pressure upon the nerves require time to return to their original position. The result is that you probably will need a number of chiropractic treatments before your ligaments finally hold your vertebrae in proper alignment.

During the healing process your body works backwards from your present state though the various intermediate states to where you were originally healthy. Thus, symptoms you had on your downward journey may show up as your body retraces its steps back to vibrant health. This retracing/healing process typically takes time. It seems that the retracing episodes follow a very measurable schedule; 1 - 2 weeks, 5 - 6 weeks, 3 months, 6 months, 9 months, and 12 months being the most noticeable.

In acute cases, these retracing symptoms may be so slight that you may not notice them. However, with chronic conditions, if your vertebrae are quickly returned to their normal positions, an entire series of symptoms may develop at one time. Thus, you may think you are getting worse, not better and stop the chiropractic treatments. Yet it is at this very time that you need to continue with chiropractic care because good things are happening—your body is retracing its steps and healing itself as it progresses.[12]

Will Upper Cervical Spine Treatment Help You?

The short answer is, "most likely", but you won't know for sure until you have tried this treatment. Here are some common ear and related questions that may indicate your atlas is "off", and thus you could benefit from upper cervical chiropractic treatments.

1. Do you have ear symptoms such as tinnitus, watery sounds in your ear, your ears feel blocked, or you have Ménière's Disease, otalgia (ear pain), or recurrent ear infections?

2. Do you often get headaches or migraines?

3. Can you remember any trauma (even minor) to your head, neck or shoulders?

4. Do you experience any balance problems such as dizziness, vertigo or movement sensations when nothing is moving?

If you answered yes to one or more of these questions, it might be wise to get yourself checked out by an upper cervical chiropractor.[13]

Finding an Upper Cervical Chiropractor

By now you probably are eager to find an upper cervical chiropractor and see what they can do to help you bring your Ménière's disease under control. Fortunately, upper cervical chiropractors are easy to find if you know where to look.

Greg Buchanan's website, (http://www.upcspine.com) gives a wealth of information on upper cervical chiropractic. Furthermore, he maintains a list of upper cervical chiropractors scattered all over the world so you (hopefully) can find one near you. Just go to the above link and click on the fifth button across the top "Practitioners". From the drop-down menu choose your area of the world. If you live in the USA or Canada, choose North America, then click on the "View" button (on the right) for your state (or province) and you will see an alphabetic listing (by chiropractor's last names—not business names) of the upper cervical chiropractors in that state/province. Each listing gives not only all the contact information you need, but also what method of upper cervical techniques they use, what instruments they use, whether they take X-rays or not, etc.

You can also go to the main web page for each of the various upper cervical chiropractic associations (each organization is associated with one specific method) and look at the listing of chiropractors trained in their method. These listings may be more complete and up-to-date than those on Buchanan's website so it's wise to check out both.

To find an upper cervical chiropractor that practices a specific method (such as the Blair method), go to Buchanan's web page that lists these various methods (http://www.upcspine.com/tech.htm) and click on the name of the method you want to investigate (in the column on the left) or on the "Read More" link at the bottom of the paragraph describing the method on the main part of the page. Usually there is a listing of chiropractors using that method somewhere on that website.

Look for upper cervical chiropractors that have/do the following:

1. A good number of years of experience (a minimum of 15 or 20 years). This is because it takes years of practicing to become an **expert** upper cervical chiropractor, especially in treating a complex condition such as Ménière's disease.

2. A chiropractor that uses the Blair method (if you can find one reasonably close to you).

3. A chiropractor that has a proven track record in successfully treating people with Ménière's disease.

4. A chiropractor that uses at least two methods to tell if you are in proper alignment (X-rays and thermography, for example).

5. A chiropractor that takes X-rays so he won't miss tiny subluxations.

If you want to start with the most experienced upper cervical chiropractor for Ménière's disease and other difficult neurological cases, you can't go wrong by contacting Dr. Burcon's clinic. He has a spectacular 97% success rate for people with Ménière's disease and trigeminal neuralgia.[14] He treats people from all over the world (and also sometimes collaborates with an upper cervical chiropractor near you if you need extended treatment).

Dr. Burcon's contact information is on his website at http://www.burconchiropractic.com. Select "Contact" (on the left). Also, check out the "Burcon Chiropractic Research Institute" website at http://www.iahp.com/BurconChiropracticcom/ for further information about him.

Last, but certainly not least, don't forget to investigate each chiropractor before you commit to him/her (some chiropractors are better than others, some have more training than others, some have more experience with Ménière's than others, some have better testing protocols than other, etc.). You alone are responsible for your own health, so do your own "due diligence", then decide whether you want to proceed, and if you choose to proceed, to whom you want to go.

Yes, It Really Works—Leon's Story

Upper cervical chiropractic treatments really work. Here is Leon's story.

> I am 64 years old. Up until three years ago when I was diagnosed with it, I had never heard of Ménière's disease. In the summer of 2012, I had a major textbook drop attack: muscle failure, intense vertigo, profuse sweating and violent vomiting. From then on, I was averaging two attacks a week. I am 5' 9" tall, and in a period of eight months, I went from 160 - 165 pounds down to 145 pounds. I was almost unable to work. In hindsight, I had been having drop attacks without the vomiting since my mid-30s. I always assumed that it was stress and blood-sugar related.
>
> In February, 2015, Dr. Neil Bauman released his article, "Atlas Adjustments Alleviate Ménière's Disease". His report caught my attention.

On March 19, 2015, I went to visit a chiropractor, who, after taking X-rays and other assessments—three hours worth—determined that my top vertebra, (C_1 or Atlas) was indeed "out" so he put it back "in". At that time, he had had approximately 15 to 20 Ménière's patients, all of whom had reductions in their vertigo and related symptoms after treatment.

The afternoon of my first visit I felt different inside—an indefinable improvement in my general inner self.

Pressure in my ears and fullness in my head had always been a constant. On Day 2, my ears started occasionally popping. On Day 3, I blew my nose and my left ear exploded in multiple pops! It felt as though I was blowing mucus right out of my ear, followed by a very pleasant empty feeling.

My feet have been numb between my toes and upper pad for approximately 4 to 5 years now. On Day 3, I noticed that my right foot was no longer numb!

My tinnitus is louder or softer at times, but has been constantly with me for the last 40 years. Occasionally I will hear five different simultaneous pitches from sleigh bells to a hammer banging on a 45-gallon drum. On Day 4 while driving home from work, I suddenly noticed that there was no ringing that I could hear. In disbelief, I quickly reached up and turned off my cochlear implant. It was true. I could not hear a single tinnitus sound. It returned by evening.

Day 5 I woke up in the middle of the night because it was so quiet. No ringing again. Too quiet to sleep I guess.

Day 6 I could hear well enough with my left ear that I could talk on my cell phone! I heard other things louder than normally with the tiny bit of residual hearing that has continued to come and go from time to time since going deaf in three months in early 2013. My hearing has improved somewhat beginning last August. I never thought hearing a toilet flush would sound so beautiful! I can still talk on my cell phone to certain people occasionally.

I have begun sleeping better and have had an increase in energy.

My chiropractor informed me that many times patients experience what he refers to as a preview window. In other words, he said that I might note a reduction in my current symptoms, but this window will only last a short time. However, this will give me an idea of what I can ultimately expect as my body retraces and heals itself.

Retracing is a healing phenomenon that our bodies do. In essence, it retraces symptoms and sometimes the emotions that accompanied a certain illness, particularly a traumatic one.

I have had my share of retracing these last few weeks. However, I have not had any vertigo attacks, but I have experienced "down days".

I have not had a vertigo attack since July 2014. Up until a few weeks ago I had attributed that to herbs, water, reduced stress, etc. All of which I am sure have helped some. However, at Week 3, I remembered I had gone to our family chiropractor the previous year.

I began wondering, "What if"? "What did he do last year"? So I drove to his office and the receptionist checked that I had had two appointments in August. The chiropractor came into the reception area at that point. I asked him if he remembered what he did to me last year. His answer quite frankly blew me away! He said, "Your C_2 was out and I put it back in. That's what we do for people with Ménière's".

Another thought occurred to me just two weeks ago. I remembered, "When I was 20, a group of us were playing football on an asphalt parking lot. I went out for a pass while running full speed and watching the ball. I turned my head to check my path, and instantly ran into a metal light pole. I remember hearing a distinct "Bing" as I hit it. I was knocked out cold. It never once occurred to me that hitting that pole with my body already turned at an angle caused my upper vertebrae to be knocked out of place. Furthermore, I certainly never considered that incident as likely being the underlying cause for my Ménière's with all of the accompanying symptoms.

On my second visit to my upper cervical chiropractor, he asked me about any improvement with my hearing. It seems that improved hearing occurs frequently. On the downside, I asked about tinnitus and he said that seems to be the last symptom to go. Overall, he has had improved hearing and reduced tinnitus in 60% of his Ménière's patients.

It is now Month 9 of the retracing of the C_1 vertebra. Month 9 is generally the most severe retracing period, and I've not been looking forward to it. So far, the only symptoms since Month 5 have been constant ringing and once feeling that unmistakable feeling of terror just before an attack, but it never came through. The hearing in my left, non-cochlear-implanted ear has come back enough that I think with a really strong hearing aid I could hear with it.

———

Today marks one full year since having my C_1 vertebra realigned. Thank you Dr. Neil for posting your report. It has changed my life.

As I mentioned, I have not had a Ménière's drop attack since July 2014 when my local chiropractor put my C_2 put back in place, nor have I had an attack of vertigo whatsoever since having my C_1 vertebra put back in place one year ago today.

Note: It is essential in most instances to periodically and regularly return to your chiropractor to ensure that your vertebrae are still in place. At this point, it appears that my C_1 vertebra has remained in place, although my C_2 may have dislodged once, but was immediately put back in. I've been back approximately 10 to 15 times for treatments this past year.

I am now able to work a full day with no trouble. I've experienced "retracing" or healing episodes, but I have not had any drop attacks or even bona fide vertigo since.

After having his vertebrae "out" for approximately 45 years, Leon is now almost back to normal after just one year. This can be your experience too, if you, like Leon, go to a good upper cervical spine chiropractor and get your head "screwed on straight". Then you can finally kiss good bye to your Ménière's (and other) symptoms that have plagued you for so long.

Other Treatments

Once an upper cervical chiropractor has properly aligned your upper cervical vertebrae, then, if you still have some symptoms of Ménière's disease, you may choose to look at some of the other treatments that people used before they knew about upper cervical spine treatments. Depending on the exact cause of your Ménière's, certain of these treatments may be more effective than others.

Teetering on the Edge of the Ménière's Precipice

Although the fundamental cause of Ménière's, as we now know, is the C_1 and C_2 vertebrae being out of alignment and putting pressure on the 5th, 7th and 8th cranial nerves, the following treatments sometimes seem to help some people to some degree, and other times not. Why?

I liken it to teetering on a fence set at the edge of a precipice. You are right at the tipping point. You can easily fall off either way depending which way an eddy of wind catches you. Anything that pushes you back from the edge so you fall off on the safe side is good. However, it doesn't take much to push you the other way and you fall over the precipice and down you go.

Thus, even little changes can make the difference whether you get a Ménière's attack or not, or how bad it is, or how long it lasts, but these little changes don't alter the fact that you still fundamentally have Ménière's disease.

That is why acupuncture or extra sleep or eating regularly might push you back from the edge, while extra salt or caffeine or stress might push you over the edge.

Therefore, even though your C_1 and C_2 vertebrae may be "out", there are a number of things you can do that may help reduce both the incidence and the severity of your Ménière's attacks (although it seems the height of foolishness to teeter on the brink of the Ménière's precipice, when you could be safely on solid ground by seeking treatment from an good upper cervical spine chiropractor).

Over the years, doctors have tried many different treatments on people with Ménière's disease. Some treatments work fairly well for some people. Other treatments are not effective, although people may believe in them. Perhaps these treatments have a placebo effect.

The truth is that no given treatment works for everyone, yet every treatment seems to work for someone. Therefore, after your neck has been properly aligned, if you need further help, investigate which treatment or treatments might work for you.

Following are a number of different treatment protocols that have worked for various people with Ménière's disease. The order of these treatment protocols begins with the easiest and least invasive (most conservative) treatments first, and progresses through more invasive and riskier treatments towards the end.

Do Nothing—Let Nature Take Its Course

If you have Ménière's disease, you can choose to do nothing and wait until the attacks pass. Some people can have several attacks that disable them for several months, and then the attacks disappear as suddenly as they began—all without them doing anything.

Your Ménière's disease may spontaneously go into remission for days, weeks, months or years. If that happens, be thankful. There is no way to predict whether this will happen to you, and, if it does happen to you, how long the remission will last.

Studies show that if you do nothing there is a 50% chance that your vertigo will disappear on its own within 2 years and a 71% chance that it will be completely gone after 8 years. This is not because your balance system has recovered and returned to normal, but because it has been irreversibly damaged and no longer functions.[15] Unfortunately, your tinnitus and hearing loss will still remain.

However, if you have more severe Ménière's attacks, you will likely want to try some of the following treatments to help alleviate the horrible vertigo you are experiencing.

Natural Healing—Visit a Naturopathic Doctor (ND)

If your health is not what you want it to be, including your Ménière's disease, you might want to do what Amy did and visit a naturopathic physician. She explained,

> There were several different things that helped me, but all of them were important.
>
> First, I went through a process to see if I was allergic to anything, and what foods triggered my Ménière's disease. I found salt is a big one; so is any form of caffeine including chocolate; alcohol; anything with nitrates in it; and some cheeses that have been aged.
>
> The most important trigger for me was not having the right amount of sleep. So too, was not eating on a normal schedule.
>
> The naturopath put me on B vitamins. She found I was low in magnesium, phosphorus, potassium, and the B vitamins. I take the magnesium with calcium when I have an attack. It helps to calm me down and relaxes my muscles. I tend to get tense in my shoulders and then I know I will have a very bad attack shortly. Smaller attacks do not do that.

Notice that in Amy's case, her Ménière's attacks come on when she feels tightness building up in her shoulders and neck. This is exactly the place where the vertebrae are that cause Ménière's disease in the first place.

Amy continues,

> My prescription now for Ménière's from the naturopath is taking B100, calcium/magnesium as needed, phosphorus as needed, vitamin D_3, drinking a lot of water—several glasses throughout the day, eating on a regular schedule with very limited salt, eight hours of sleep a day (and more if Ménière's attacks cause me to need more sleep) and the least amount of stress possible, including not working more than one job.
>
> Acupuncture as needed. I did one session every week for 6 to 8 weeks. It helped a lot. My naturopath told me acupuncture works for some people but not for others. The acupuncture started working after 3 to 4 weeks of needles behind my ears. I had a lot of fluid behind my ears so that was the only needle that hurt due to the pressure against my balance and hearing nerves. It got better the more I did the acupuncture. Massage also helps with my tension. I still have bad days but it is 80% better than before.

Thus, you would do well to be checked out by a naturopathic doctor. Not only will you have a good chance of improving your health, but you may also alleviate your Ménière's symptoms as well.

Avoid or Eliminate Triggers for Ménière's Attacks

Once you have Ménière's disease, there are any number of things that may seem to trigger further Ménière's attacks. Note that triggers do not cause Ménière's disease—that is due to your C_1 and C_2 vertebrae being out of proper alignment. Rather, triggers are things that can induce or exacerbate your existing Ménière's symptoms. These triggers vary greatly from person to person. No one trigger affects all people. You might have a trigger that no one else has, or you might not have as a trigger something that affects many people with Ménière's disease. However, there are a number of triggers that are common to numbers of people with Ménière's disease.

When it comes right down to it, if you have Ménière's disease, you don't really care what things trigger attacks in other people. You want to know what things specifically trigger attacks in your case; then you want to learn how to either eliminate those triggers or avoid setting off those triggers in the future.

There are three general categories of Ménière's triggers—food triggers, environmental triggers and lifestyle triggers.

Food Triggers

Salt: Most doctors agree that the number one trigger of Ménière's disease is too much sodium in your diet. Sodium causes your body to retain fluid. It is excess fluid in your body that doctors typically think causes excess endolymph to build up in your inner ears, resulting in Ménière's attacks. (For more information on salt and Ménière's, see point 2 in "Dietary Changes" below.)

Trans-Fats: A diet high in trans-fats may also cause Ménière's attacks by clogging up your arteries with cholesterol. By obstructing blood flow to your ears, you may trigger Ménière's attacks.

Sugar: Eating too many sweet foods—foods high in sugar can also bring on Ménière's attacks. (For more information on sugar and Ménière's, see point 3 in "Dietary Changes" below.)

Caffeine: Too much caffeine causes Ménière's attacks in some people. Caffeine is commonly found in coffee, tea, colas, chocolate and some drugs. (For more information on caffeine and Ménière's, see point 4 in "Dietary Changes" below.)

Chocolate: Some people find that eating chocolate triggers their Ménière's attacks. The root cause may be the sugar and caffeine in the chocolate.

Alcohol: Drinking alcohol is another common Ménière's trigger. (For more information on alcohol and Ménière's, see point 6 in "Dietary Changes" below.)

Environmental Triggers

Barometric pressure: There seems to be a correlation between barometric pressure and the onset of Ménière's attacks in some people. As Dr. Salt explained,

> I have heard many patients report that pressure changes can make symptoms worse, whether it is from driving up a mountain, the passing of a weather front or the pressure changes that occur during flying.[16]

Many people complain that heavy, damp weather tends to spark their Ménière's attacks. One person reported,

> I have noticed that during days when the air is "heavy" I tend to have more symptoms.

Another lady with similar experiences remarked,

> For me it can be caused by barometric pressure changes—when the air pressure is very low I feel sick, but when it gets higher (the barometer is over 30) I feel better. When a storm is coming—even up to 2 days before it hits, I can get sick.

Tom wrote,

> I can remember many flights over the years that left me with intense pressure in my ears along with dizziness and disorientation, sometimes for days. Changes in weather are not quite as intense, but often I've thought I would make a good barometer!

Unfortunately, doctors don't seem to realize just how much small changes in air pressure can affect people with Ménière's disease. Leigh explained,

> According to my ENT doctor, changes in air pressure from storms or planes is so minimal to the inner ear that they dismiss it. I told him that every spring storm makes me spin like a top. He had a hard time wrapping his head around that. I don't trust a doctor to tell me how I'm affected when it's as clear as day to me—storms come—I'm on the floor—spinning.

Allergies: Air-borne allergies, sinus infections and hay fever all seem to trigger Ménière's attacks in some people. Other people are very sensitive to all kinds of mold, which triggers their Ménière's attacks. (For more information on allergies and Ménière's, see "Allergy treatments" below.)

Chemicals: Some people are sensitive to common household cleaners and pesticides, or to various chemicals used in industry.

Personal and Lifestyle Triggers

Smoking: For a number of people smoking triggers their Ménière's attacks. As a result, most doctors advise people with Ménière's disease to cut out smoking.

Stress: High levels of stress, or prolonged stress, can trigger Ménière's attacks. (For more information on stress reduction as it relates to Ménière's disease, see "Stress Reduction" below.)

Lack of sleep: Overtiredness and lack of sleep can bring on Ménière's attacks. If you have Ménière's disease, you need adequate sleep and rest. As Pam explained, "I know that lack of sleep really seems to bring on attacks for me."

Bright or flashing lights: For some people bright or flashing lights, or moving lights such as occurs when you are driving at night, can trigger Ménière's attacks.

Rapid eye or head movements: Quick movements of the head or eyes can bring on Ménière's attacks, particularly if your vestibular system is already damaged.

Eye glasses: Eye glasses that are not the right prescription can trigger Ménière's attacks in some people. So can wearing bifocals. As one lady explained,

> It is better for me to have separate reading and regular glasses. Transitional lens are the best for moving from dark to light places (i.e. for going outside).

Visual problems while moving: For some people reading while moving, e.g. reading while riding in a moving vehicle or train, or while flying, can trigger Ménière's attacks. Problems can also arise when watching horizontal movement in movies or on the TV, or when walking down a visually "busy" supermarket aisle. For some people, the trigger is vertical parallel lines while moving, such as riding down streets lined with telephone poles, fence posts, guard rail posts, or trees.

Monthly periods: Some women find that their Ménière's attacks are associated with their monthly periods.

Migraine headaches: For numbers of people there is an association between their migraine headaches and their Ménière's attacks.

This gives you an idea of some of the many things that can trigger Ménière's attacks in people, but it is not an exhaustive list. If you can identify and avoid the triggers that cause your Ménière's attacks, you can likely reduce the frequency and/or severity of succeeding Ménière's attacks. As a result, it may be worth your while to search out and eliminate any triggers you find that cause your Ménière's attacks.

Dietary Changes

Once you are diagnosed with Ménière's disease, the first treatment doctors typically suggest is that you change your diet. The good news is that if you strictly adhere to an appropriate dietary regimen, you will very likely see some reduction in the severity of your Ménière's symptoms.

The reason for this is that when your body is working normally, the fluid-filled balance mechanisms in your inner ears operate **independently** of your body's fluid/blood system. Your body maintains the proper fluid pressure in your inner ears, and also maintains the proper concentration of electrolytes such as sodium, potassium, chloride, etc. When something goes wrong, such as happens when you have Ménière's disease, your body loses this independent control. The result is that the fluid pressure and electrolyte concentrations in your inner ears vary in step with changes to your body's fluid/blood.

The trick is to keep your body's fluid/blood concentration of salt (sodium) and sugar relatively constant. This limits the resulting fluctuations in the fluids in your inner ears and minimizes the symptoms of Ménière's disease.

How can you do this? The Vestibular Disorders Association (VEDA) recommends the following dietary guidelines.[17] Of course, you want to do this under the care of a qualified health-care professional.

1. Distribute your food and fluid intake evenly throughout the day, and from day to day. Eat approximately the same amount of food at each meal. Do not skip meals. If you have snacks, have them at the same time each day.

2. Severely limit the amount of sodium in your diet. The most common source of sodium is table salt (sodium chloride). Therefore, you typically need to greatly reduce your salt intake. In addition to the salt you add to your food, you will have to watch for the hidden salt that most packaged and prepared foods contain. High salt levels in your diet will result in increased pressure in your inner ears, which you want to avoid. Aim for a diet that is high in fresh fruits, vegetables and whole grains. Limit your intake of canned, frozen and processed foods as these often contain the most salt.

   Typically you should limit your sodium intake to 1½ to 2 grams (1,500 mg to 2,000 mg) per day.[18,19] Some people with Ménière's try to limit their sodium intake to between 500 and 1,000 mg per day, but that is extreme. Dr. Hain explains,

   > It is not necessary, or wise, to lower your salt intake to amounts barely able to sustain life. We do not encourage 1 gram [1,000 mg] sodium diets. Rather, the goal is to keep sodium levels from fluctuating. A 2-gram [2,000 mg] diet is usually possible.[20]

   Note: this is not a 2-gram **salt** diet—but rather a 2-gram **sodium** diet. Salt has both sodium and chlorine. You only need to control the sodium part. For your information, one teaspoon of table salt equals about 2 grams of sodium.

The hope is that by limiting the amount of salt in your diet, and thus the overall amount of fluid in your body, the amount of endolymph will also reduce in the process.

Some people find a strong correlation between their salt intake and their Ménière's symptoms. Other people don't seem to find any correlation at all. Alan explained,

> As far as diet goes, salt was the main factor for me. I went on a low sodium diet. My wife even made bread that was sodium free. My diet was reviewed by a dietician at one point, and she could not think of any way to reduce my sodium intake further. If I did consume sodium, I could feel it within hours: my tinnitus increased, my disequilibrium would increase and maybe lead to vertigo, and my hearing seemed to decline a bit. I guess that quick response was one of the things that helped me get off sodium as much as possible. I could see a cause and effect relationship.

Researchers have found some correlation between salt intake and certain hormone levels in your body that, in turn, affect the way your body regulates endolymph.

> **Low-sodium Diet Recipes**
>
> The Low Sodium Cooking website (http://www.lowsodiumcooking.com) contains many tasty, low-sodium recipes. In addition, it gives sources for low sodium cookbooks, etc.

Incidentally, a recent study found a correlation between airsickness and sodium intake—the more salt in your diet, the more you get airsick.[21]

3. Severely limit the amount of sugar in your diet. In addition to the sugar you add to your food, you will have to watch for the hidden sugars that most packaged and prepared foods contain. High sugar levels in your diet will result in increased pressure in your inner ears, which you want to avoid. Aim for a diet that is high in fresh fruits, vegetables and whole grains. Limit your intake of canned, frozen and processed foods as these often contain the most sugar.

   High sugar levels and foods with a high glycemic index can bring on Ménière's-like symptoms, or make your existing Ménière's worse. Penny explained,

> I've been grappling with a lot of tinnitus lately and my hearing has been fluctuating to extremes. I've been close to being deaf with terribly muffled sounds. I went to see Dr Derebery [at the House Clinic in Los Angeles, CA] recently, and we talked about my eating habits, and the fact that I wake up every 3 hours at night with my head pounding. I have to eat something to get it to stop so I can sleep again.
>
> The thing is, I would eat cereal with rice milk and raw sugar. Dr. Derebery suggested I could be hypoglycemic. She put me on the hypoglycemic diet, which means no sugar at all, no rice, no pasta, no corn, etc, but lots of protein, eating regularly with snacks between meals, etc. The **first day** on this diet my tinnitus stopped completely. I started sleeping through the night. My hearing has cleared up big time. She said that sugar is the most difficult substance for the ear to deal with.

4. Eliminate caffeine (coffee, tea, colas, chocolate, and even some drugs)[22] from your diet. Caffeine is both a diuretic and a stimulant. Because of this, taking it may bring on an attack or make your existing symptoms worse. Numerous Ménière's sufferers have reported attacks within minutes of using caffeine.[23] For others, caffeine has no effect on their Ménière's attacks. Caffeine can also make your tinnitus worse. In addition, you should know that ingesting large amounts of caffeine may trigger migraine headaches. These headaches may trigger (or mimic) Ménière's attacks.

5. Drink adequate amounts of fluids each day (5 to 7 glasses)[24] such as water, milk and low-sugar fruit juices (e.g. cranberry or cranapple juice). However, be cautious about drinking milk. You may have an allergy to milk and thus get Ménière's/allergy symptoms from milk and milk products. If you anticipate losing excess fluid because of heat or exercise, replace these fluids **before** they are lost.

6. Cut out alcohol since it changes both the volume and concentration of the fluids in your inner ears. Again, this results in increased Ménière's symptoms in some people, but not in others. In fact, alcohol can be a massive trigger of Ménière's attacks in some people, and yet doesn't seem to be a factor with others. Alcohol may also trigger migraine-associated vertigo.[25]

   Alcohol acts differently with different people. For some people the Ménière's attacks come while they are still drinking; for others the attacks come shortly after they have finished drinking; and for still others, the attacks occur the next day. For example, "Andy" found that after drinking alcohol, something rather peculiar happened. It improved his balance for a few hours, but his balance was worse the next day or the day after. For Alan, alcohol had a beneficial effect. He explained,

> I noticed that when I'd come home from work and have a glass of wine or two I'd feel better—less disequilibrium, but it did not affect my balance the next day. One of my ENTs said that was because of the tranquilizing effect of the alcohol in the wine.

Incidentally, beer can cause a double whammy for people with Ménière's disease as it not only contains alcohol, but also often contains considerable amounts of salt.

7. Avoid foods containing MSG (monosodium glutamate) as it is very high in sodium. MSG is often found in Chinese food and in some packaged foods.

8. Avoid *Aspirin* and medications containing it. *Aspirin* can increase both your tinnitus and your dizziness. Also, avoid any other medications that affect your ears.

    Alan explains,

> Some common drugs are known to be toxic to the inner ear. Most people are not bothered by them. However, they can affect those of us who are prone to disequilibrium and vertigo. Some people have a link between their balance episodes and things such as Ibuprofen, Acetaminophen (*Tylenol*) *Aspirin* and Naproxen. If I take one of those at night, the next day I will feel off-kilter till about noon, when things seem to go back to my normal state of balance. For me, the most pronounced effect is brought on by Ibuprofen and Naproxen, less so with *Tylenol* or *Aspirin*. I also find that most antihistamines have a negative effect on me in terms of balance. So too, does tonic water, which contains quinine. In fact, drinking a single gin and tonic on the rare occasion I have one has a greater impact on my equilibrium and tinnitus the next day than do most of the pain medications.

Ototoxic Drugs

Our book *Ototoxic Drugs Exposed* contains the details of 877 drugs known to affect/damage people's ears. See the back of this book for further information.

9. If you are a smoker, stop smoking. Nicotine is toxic to your inner ears. Nicotine also constricts your blood vessels, thus decreasing the blood

supply to your inner ears. This can make your symptoms worse and make these other suggestions ineffective.[26,27]

10. You may want to increase your potassium intake, especially if you are on water pills (diuretics).[28] Good sources of potassium include bananas, cantaloupe, dried fruits, navy beans, nectarines, orange juice, potatoes, raisins, unsalted peanuts and winter squash.[29]

11. If you are into complementary or alternative medicine, you might want to consider taking Ginkgo biloba, a vasodilator, which also increases blood flow to your ears, and/or Vinpocetine—a compound derived from the lesser Periwinkle plant (Vinca minor)—which increases blood circulation in your brain. Some people with Ménière's find it helps them.

12. A number of Ménière's sufferers find that taking Ginger root (Zingiber officinale) helps to reduce their nausea.

13. Consider taking Vitamin B_3 (Niacin/Nicotinic acid). Niacin increases peripheral vascular blood flow, which is a fancy way of saying it increases blood flow to your inner ears. Pam explained,

    > I was told by a friend of mine, who also struggled with Ménière's, to try taking Niacin every day, and that had helped him to stop having attacks for 7 years. I was skeptical, but I tried it, and I have not had one of those "emergency room all day" types of attacks in several months now. My "dizzies" still come and go, but they are not as bad as they were before.

Your body is unique in how it reacts to dietary changes and restrictions. What works for one person may not work for you (and vice versa). So, for example, if you try eliminating caffeine from your diet and it makes no difference to your Ménière's attacks, maybe your Ménière's is not affected by caffeine. Therefore, you may decide to resume drinking coffee, whereas another person may have violent Ménière's attacks each time they drink a cup of coffee. This is just the way it is. As a result, you have to experiment on yourself and see what works for you. When you find a food strategy that reduces the frequency or intensity of your attacks, then, by all means, continue using that strategy.

Boost Your Immune System

If your Ménière's symptoms are the result of underlying problems with your immune system (and as explained previously, many doctors are now coming to this conclusion), one approach is to rebalance your immune system in order to gain control over your Ménière's symptoms. (Remember, as we saw previously, that when your C_1 and C_2 vertebrae are out of proper alignment, this can affect the proper functioning of your immune system so keep this in mind as you read the following.)

When you have autoimmune problems, your immune system is obviously "out of whack". Therefore, you want to regulate your immune system and bring it into proper balance again. In order to do this, typically you need to improve your body's immune system T-cell function, while at the same time reducing its over-active B-cell activity. The natural way to do this is to enhance your body's ability to produce adequate amounts of glutathione (gloo-tah-THIGH-own).[30]

Research has shown that the immune cells of people with autoimmune diseases are typically deficient in glutathione, the body's powerful natural antioxidant. Glutathione not only is a powerful antioxidant, but also is critical to helping keep your immune system working properly, and in detoxifying your body.[31]

Researchers in both Japan and Italy have shown significant improvement in Ménière's symptoms (vertigo, tinnitus and hearing loss) by raising the body's overall level of glutathione. In one study of 22 people with Ménière's disease, 21 (95%) showed marked improvement in vertigo, 12 (55%) showed improvement in hearing and 18 (82%) showed improvement in tinnitus.[32]

Since glutathione is not well absorbed by the stomach, taking glutathione supplements doesn't work well. A better approach is to provide your body with the proper nutritional pre-cursors it needs to produce glutathione. Since glutathione is a combination of three amino acids—cysteine, glycine and glutamine—you should take foods and supplements high in these substances.

Foods that support glutathione production include garlic, onions, broccoli, kale, collards, cabbage, cauliflower; watercress, etc.[33]

Supplement these foods with one of the main building blocks of glutathione, namely N-acetyl-cysteine. In addition, take alpha lipoic acid; the antioxidant Vitamins C and E; the mineral, selenium; and the herbal, milk thistle (Silybum marianum).

At the same time, don't forget to take Vitamins B_6, B_9 and B_{12}. According to Dr. Hyman, these are critical to keeping your body producing glutathione. (Incidentally, it is best to take the active forms of these three vitamins. Thus, for Vitamin B_6—pyridoxine—the active form is P5P [pyridoxal-5-phosphate]; for Vitamin B_9—folic acid or folate—the active form is 5-methyltetrahydrofolate; and for Vitamin B_{12} the active form is methylcobalamin.)[34]

Finally, don't forget to exercise to boost your glutathione levels—30 minutes a day of walking or jogging should suffice.[35]

Stress Reduction

Stress can trigger Ménière's attacks. This happens to numbers of people with Ménière's disease. Along with many others, Marty echoes, "For me it is tension and stress". Stress could be from overwork, for example, or emotional distress. According to Dr. Gibson, often people who suffer with Ménière's disease like neatness and order in their lives. When their lives become too busy, or when problems arise, this causes them undue stress. As a result, they may experience Ménière's attacks.[36] Sometimes the Ménière's attacks come just **after** the stress has abated. Marty adds,

> I have found that many times I get hit by a Ménière's attack **after** the stress is over. For some reason I get through the stressful period, but once I relax again, I get hit hard.

Note: stress can show up in other symptoms. For example, if you have temporomandibular disorders (TMD) (tight jaw/pain in jaw) and cervical spine disorders (CSD) (tight neck/pain in neck) as well as Ménière's disease, that is a strong indication your upper cervical spine is out of alignment and you should seek out an upper cervical spine chiropractor to get your back properly aligned again

In one study, the results of coordinated treatments showed "simultaneous decreases in the intensities of vertigo, non-whirling dizziness, tinnitus, feeling of fullness in the ear, pain in the face and jaw, pain in the neck and shoulders, and headaches which were statistically highly significant. In addition, there were significant reductions in vertigo, non-whirling dizziness and headaches, as well as the complete disappearance of pain in the vertex area [top back part of the head].

As you have seen previously, and as these results prove, Ménière's disease has a clear association with both TMD and CSD (specifically C_1 and C_2 being out of alignment) and is made worse by stress, nervousness and muscular tension."[37]

If your Ménière's attacks are related to stress, you need to learn how to get your stress under control, and how to avoid stressful situations as much as possible so your body doesn't "tighten up". Doing so can reduce the incidence and severity of your Ménière's attacks.

Medications for Ménière's

Doctors prescribe a number of drugs to treat Ménière's disease—mostly to control the vertigo and nausea that so often accompanies it. The good news is that with proper medication it is possible to control, or at least lessen, the nausea, vomiting, and vertigo about 70 to 90 percent of the time.

Drug therapy can be divided into four main groups to treat various Ménière's symptoms. Some of the more common drugs in each group are shown below.

Key to Drugs Mentioned Here

Bold	Generic name of an ototoxic drug (e.g. **Meclizine**).
Regular	Generic name of a drug not known to be ototoxic (e.g. Prochlorperazine).
Italics	Brand name of a generic drug (e.g. *Antivert*).
Small Capitals	Drug Classes (e.g. Benzodiazepines).

Vestibular Suppressants

Doctors prescribe vestibular suppressants to reduce the severity of acute vertigo attacks.

- Antihistamines (Piperazines) such as:
    - **Meclizine** (*Antivert*).
    - **Cinnarizine** (*Stugeron*).
    - **Flunarizine (*Sibelium*).** Note that both Cinnarizine and Flunarizine are commonly used in the UK, but not in the USA.[38]
    - **Betahistine** (*Serc*) is used extensively in the UK as a vestibular suppressant for treatment of Ménière's disease. However, in the USA, the FDA has ruled that there is little evidence to prove that it works, although it is available here.
- Anti-cholinergic drugs such as:
    - **Dimenhydrinate** (*Dramamine*).

- Benzodiazepines such as:
    - **Lorazepam** (*Ativan*).
    - **Clonazepam** (*Klonopin*).
    - **Diazepam** (*Valium*).

    The Benzodiazepines not only can reduce the severity of vertigo attacks, but also they are tranquillizers and can calm you down and reduce your anxiety so your Ménière's doesn't bother you as much.

- Calcium Channel Blockers such as:
    - **Verapamil** (*Isoptin*).
    - **Nimodipine** (*Nimotop*).

    Calcium Channel Blockers may reduce the severity and frequency of Ménière's attacks. Their main role may be to treat migraine-associated vertigo that can be confused with, or accompany, Ménière's attacks. These medications are logical if the dizzy attacks are associated with headaches.[39]

Anti-emetics

Doctors prescribe anti-emetics to control vomiting and feelings of nausea.

- **Ondansetron** (*Zofran*) is a Gastrointestinal drug (Serotonin-receptor antagonist).
- **Promethazine** (*Phenergan*) is an Antihistamine (H_1 receptor antagonist).
- **Prochlorperazine** (*Compazine, Stemetil*)[40] is a Phenothiazine.

Diuretics

If you have dizziness symptoms between acute Ménière's attacks, your doctor may prescribe diuretics (water pills). Diuretics flush excessive fluid from your body. If one doesn't work for you, try another. For some reason, certain diuretics work for one person but not for another.

According to Dr. Hain, about one-third of his patients report a good response to using diuretics, while the other two-thirds don't notice any real difference one way or the other.[41]

- **Triamterene/Hydrochlorothiazide** (*Dyazide, Maxzide*). *Dyazide* is the drug most often used in the USA.
- **Amiloride/Hydrochlorothiazide** (*Moduretic*).
- **Acetazolamide** (*Diamox*).
- **Methazolamide** (*Neptazane*) Commonly used to treat glaucoma, but is sometimes prescribed for people with Ménière's disease.

Autoimmune Suppressants—Intratympanic Steroids

For severe or intractable bilateral Ménière's disease, your doctor may prescribe intratympanic steroids—that is, steroids injected though the eardrum into the middle ear cavity—especially if your Ménière's disease appears to be caused by an underlying auto-immune condition. Since steroids are not long-lasting, this procedure needs to be done several times a year.[42] Having numerous injections through your eardrum can lead to scaring and other problems with your eardrum, so this treatment is not without risk. The results of this treatment are mixed.

For Ménière's disease caused by immune system disorders, Dr. John Shea Jr. used the drug **Dexamethasone** to greatly reduce or eliminate the Ménière's symptoms with little risk of further hearing loss.[43]

In one small study of 11 people and 11 controls, of those that had the **Dexamethasone** injections, 9 gained complete control of their vertigo while the remaining 2 gained substantial control whereas, of those in the control group, 4 gained complete control, none gained substantial control, 3 gained lesser control and the remaining 4 were considered treatment failures.[44]

The common Glucocorticoid steroids used include:

- **Dexamethasone** (*Decadron*). Used to reduce inflammation and to suppress the immune system.
- **Methylprednisolone** (*Medrol*). [45]
- **Prednisone** (*Deltasone*).

Your doctor may also prescribe one of the following drugs to try to stop your immune system from attacking your inner ears.

- **Etanercept** (*Enbrel*) is a Tumor necrosis factor modifier drug.
- **Infliximab** (*Remicade*) is a Monoclonal antibody drug.
- **Methotrexate** (*Rheumatrex*) is an Anti-metabolite drug.

In addition to the above medications, there are many other drugs in various classes that doctors have tried on people with Ménière's disease with varying degrees of success. For example, Latanoprost (*Xalatan*), a drug used in the treatment of glaucoma in one study reported a 30% reduction in vertigo.

Allergy Treatments

If your Ménière's attacks are related to allergies, then you should seek out treatment for any allergies you might have. Dr. Jennifer Derebery (pronounced Deerberry) of the House Clinic in Los Angeles, CA is the expert on Ménière's disease and allergies. She holds sub-specialties in both otology and allergies. Dr. Derebery says statistics indicate that about 15 to 20 percent of Ménière's patients have allergy sensitivities, although she believes the true figure is higher. She feels that some Ménière's attacks may actually be an adult manifestation of a childhood allergy.

Incidentally, if you have Ménière's disease in both ears, there is a good chance that your Ménière's is indeed related to allergies.[46]

Both food and inhaled allergens may cause Ménière's symptoms. As in regular allergies, cutting out foods that cause your allergies is the best treatment for Ménière's symptoms produced by food allergens. Dr. Derebery says that the most common foods that produce Ménière's symptoms are wheat, corn and milk. Other foods such as beer, chocolate, red wine and shellfish can also cause Ménière's attacks.[47] If the source of the allergy is airborne, she treats the person with allergy shots, much as severe hay fever is treated.[48]

Here's an example of her treatment results. James, after years of suffering silently from Ménière's disease, heard about Dr. Derebery. She tested him for allergies and turned up several. Medication, including weekly allergy injections and diet modification, now helps keep James' Ménière's under control. When he goes out, James avoids certain foods that he knows will cause him trouble.[49]

Penny also finds that her allergies can cause Ménière's-like symptoms. She recounted,

> I never had vertigo until I moved into the house I now own. Two months after moving in, I was falling down with vertigo, crawling and puking, being flattened for hours with the world spinning. This went on for several years until one day I had a terrible attack in the waiting room at the House Clinic.
>
> Dr. Derebery told me they had just gotten new carpeting in there and that's what was causing my attack. This made me wonder about the old carpeting in my new home. I started having the old carpeting removed and found solid black mold under the carpeting in the family room. Once carpets and mold were removed the vertigo left, and I've never had a vertigo attack since, and that's over 6 years now. I have an allergy to mold. That's how severely our allergies can trigger our Ménière's symptoms.

Anti-emetic Devices

Ménière's sufferers who often experience disequilibrium such that they have a lot of nausea (and vomiting) may be interested in a non-invasive, anti-emetic device that helps people with motion sickness. When using this device, you gain relief from your nausea much as you would from taking the anti-emetic drug **Meclizine**, but without the drug's side effects.

Reliefband

The Reliefband is used for reducing nausea and vomiting from conditions such as motion sickness, morning sickness during pregnancy, nausea caused by chemotherapy and post-operative nausea.

This device, about the size of a man's wrist watch, is worn on the underside of your wrist. When you have this wrist band positioned correctly two finger widths below the first crease on your wrist, and between the two tendons, you feel a gentle pulsing or tingling sensation in your palm and/or the middle fingers of your hand every four seconds.

The Reliefband uses transdermal neuromodulation technology to stimulate the median nerve on the underside of your wrist. These electrical neural impulses travel up the median nerve to the emetic center in your brain.

The theory is that once the neural signals reach the emetic center, they act to positively modulate the various anti-nausea and vomiting feedback mechanisms and neural pathways, thus restoring the gastric rhythms in your stomach back to normal (via modulation of the vagus nerve). By positively modulating these control systems, the Reliefband uses the body's own natural neural control pathways to relieve symptoms of nausea.

The Reliefband allows you to take control of your nausea. You simply turn on the device and set it to one of five stimulation levels for fast relief when you feel nausea coming on. When your symptoms subside, you turn the device off until you need it again.

Although it was not specifically designed for people with Ménière's disease, nor is it FDA approved for that purpose, the Reliefband gives relief to some people with nausea resulting from their Ménière's attacks. For example, Jenny explained,

> I bought the Reliefband and am wearing it all day and night to help with my dizziness and vertigo. I actually sleep without being sick now. I hate to take it off when showering as all the dizziness symptoms are there the minute I take it off.

To learn more about the Reliefband, go to the Reliefband Technologies website at http://www.reliefband.com.

Positive-pressure Pulse Devices

There are a couple of positive-pressure pulse devices that may help you cope with the debilitating effects of your Ménière's attacks.

Local positive-pressure treatments are most effective in treating the symptoms of rotary vertigo due to Ménière's disease. Consequently, positive-pressure pulse treatments give the best results to those people with severe rotary vertigo—people who otherwise would be candidates for destructive surgery.

It seems that people with Ménière's disease are particularly sensitive to negative pressure in the middle ear. Researchers have known that "fluctuations in ambient pressure, like with increasing altitude, are associated with improvement in Ménière's symptoms."[50] Back in the late 1970s, researchers discovered that the symptoms of people with Ménière's disease improved when there was a relative over-pressure in the middle ear (the outside air pressure was less than the air pressure in the middle ear). They also noticed that the Ménière's symptoms worsened when there was a relative-under-pressure (the outside air pressure was higher than the air pressure in the middle ear).[51]

This led to some success in treating people having Ménière's disease attacks in hypobaric (reduced air pressure) pressure chambers. However, this was a cumbersome procedure as the person had to go to a facility that had such pressure chambers. Hyperbaric/hypobaric pressure chambers are more common in Europe, but quite rare in the USA.

This is where positive-pressure pulse treatment comes in. The idea behind this treatment is that applying positive air pressure to the middle ear would reduce the excess endolymph, and thus it would relieve the symptoms. The pressure pulses are distributed via the round window membrane to the inner ear fluids. Since the inner ear fluids are not compressible, and the membranous labyrinth is enclosed by bone, an increase in the perilymphatic pressure forces any excess endolymph out of the inner ear and into the endolymphatic duct and sac where it does not do any damage.[52]

In order to apply these positive-pressure pulses to the inner ear, your doctor must first surgically place ventilation tubes (tympanostomy tubes or grommets) in your eardrums; otherwise your eardrums would block these pressure pulses.

Incidentally, some people feel that just having ventilation tubes put in their eardrums is effective in helping reduce their Ménière's symptoms, but a number of doctors regard this procedure as a placebo.[53]

There are two positive-pressure pulse devices currently on the market. The Meniett runs on batteries. The P-100 is a manual device. Here are the details.

Meniett

The Meniett is a battery-operated low-positive-pressure pulse generator developed by Dr. Barbara Densert around 2002. Dr. Densert designed it to help control intractable vertigo in those people with Ménière's disease who are not helped by diet or diuretic drugs.

The Meniett is a pager-sized device that comes with a flexible tube and several sizes of ear tips. You select the correct size of ear tip to seal your ear canal. The device checks that you have a good seal and that the ventilation tube is still functioning properly. The Meniett has a rechargeable battery that lasts 7 to 10 days between charges with normal use (Fig. 5-1).

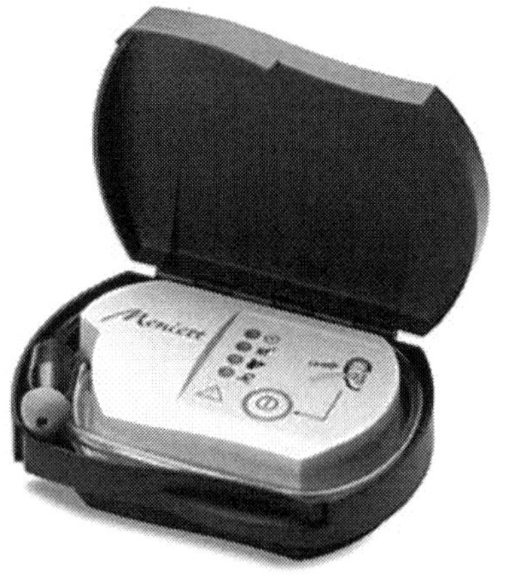

Fig. 5-1. The Meniett in its carrying case.

You give yourself three treatments per day. Each treatment consists of a 5-minute series of pulses consisting of 4 low-pressure pulses per second followed by a break of a few seconds. The Meniett repeats this cycle for 5 minutes. It indicates when the treatment sequence has successfully completed.

Don't expect instant results. When you begin using the Meniett, it can take from 1 to 3 weeks before you notice its effectiveness. However, for some people it may take as long as 5 or 6 weeks or more before they see positive results.[54]

Since your body constantly produces endolymph, and if resorption continues to be too slow, you will need to repeat this regular daily treatment indefinitely. Unless you go into remission, you will find your vertigo rapidly returns if you stop treatment.

How good is the Meniett? For people for whom low sodium diets and diuretics fail to do the job, more than 90% typically report relief when using this device.

The results of one two-year study revealed the following: 51% were now free from vertigo attacks; 41% had a significant decrease in frequency of vertigo attacks; and 8% did not respond to the Meniett treatments.

In another 2-year study, 34% of the participants went into remission, 33% were greatly improved, 9% somewhat improved, and 24% dropped out and opted for surgery to stop their vertigo.[55] That's not quite the impressive figures of the previous study, but it is still great news that 67% either went into remission or were greatly improved.

Overall, using the Meniett decreased, by about half, the number of days people with severe vertigo suffered.[56] Again, this is good news if you suffer from severe vertigo.

The Meniett is not for everyone with Ménière's disease. It is not for you if you have a perilymphatic fistula; if you have retrocochlear damage—that is, damage to the vestibulocochlear nerve or the vestibular processing parts of the brain; if you have an acoustic neuroma or brain tumor; or if you have low-pressure hydrocephalus.[57]

Currently, there are about 3,000 Ménière's sufferers using the Meniett in the USA.

The Meniett is rather pricey at $3,500.00, but if it does the job, you may think the price is worth it. Generally health insurance does not cover it, although some insurance companies cover it on a case by case basis.

You should know whether the Meniett is going to be effective for you in about 5 weeks after you begin treatment with it. The good news is that Medtronic offers you a full money-back guarantee within 6 weeks after you purchase your Meniett. Thus, if it doesn't work for you in 5 - 6 weeks, you can get your money back.[58]

Obtaining a Meniett is straightforward. If you have severe Ménière's disease, you can ask your doctor to write you a prescription for this device and FAX it to Medtronic. The company then contacts you to arrange for payment and delivery. That's it.

You can learn more about the Meniett from Medtronic Xomed in Jacksonville, FL at www.meniett.com, or contact them via their Meniett direct line at 877-966-3350.

P100—Portable Positive Pressure Pulse Therapy Device

A cheaper alternative to the Meniett is a small, hand-held device called the P100 (Fig. 5-2), made by Enttex GmbH. One study showed that the P100 gave results equal to that of the Meniett.[59]

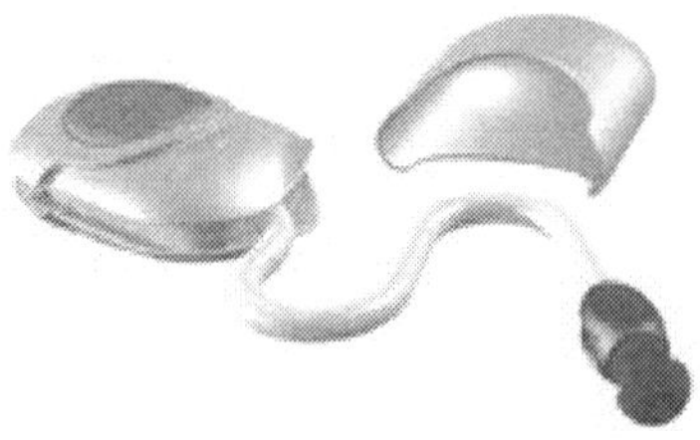

Fig. 5-2. The Enttex P100 with its cover off showing the ear tube.

As with the Meniett, before you can use this device, you have to have your doctor install pressure equalization tubes in your eardrums.

The P100 is easy to use. Just remove its protective cover, unwrap the tube and place the ear tip into your ear canal with one hand while holding the device in the other. Press the center diaphragm with your thumb to apply air pressure pulses. When you are finished, just wrap the tube around the device and replace its protective cover.

The P100 is simple and convenient to use. It doesn't require any batteries and only costs about $56.00 US. Its main disadvantage is that since it is a manual device, you have to stop what you were doing to press it to generate the pulses.

You can learn more about the P100 at the Enttex company website at http://www.enttex.eu/english/home/.

Gentamicin Injections

Another medical treatment uses **Gentamicin**, an ototoxic AMINOGLYCOSIDE antibiotic to affect the function of the vestibular (balance) system, thus eliminating the vertigo.

Doctors have known for some time that antibiotics such as **Streptomycin** and **Gentamicin** can destroy both hearing and balance. In fact, millions of people around the world owe their hearing losses to taking just such drugs in the past.

Doctors now mainly use **Gentamicin** for three reasons. First, it has a greater affinity for the tissues ("dark cells") believed responsible for endolymph production. Second, it is not as toxic as **Streptomycin**. Third, it does not have the same harmful side effects that **Streptomycin** has, such as permanent balance problems.[60]

Doctors can use **Gentamicin** in three different ways, just by varying the dose and frequency of use. Each of these ways has a different objective.

Low-dose Intratympanic Gentamicin Treatment

If you only have Ménière's disease in one ear, doctors may use a low-dose intratympanic **Gentamicin** protocol. In this treatment, your doctor injects a low dose of **Gentamicin** through the eardrum into your middle ear. The drug is left in the middle ear for about 30 minutes then allowed to drain out. This procedure is repeated twice, one month apart.

This protocol works because intratympanic **Gentamicin** injections given in very low doses can permanently affect the "dark cells" (those cells in the endolymphatic system that are thought to produce endolymph) so that they do not produce as much endolymph.

The idea is that if **Gentamicin** affects the dark cells so they can't produce as much endolymph, then there won't be an oversupply of endolymph causing the endolymphatic hydrops. With reduced endolymphatic pressure, there will be no further hearing loss or vertigo attacks. By only using the **Gentamicin** twice, the vertigo is controlled without also causing other side effects such as reduced hearing. Thus, if low-dose **Gentamicin** is used soon enough, it may preserve both hearing and balance.

The overall success rate for this protocol is about 66% to 80%, although Dr. Hain claims 100% with no reduction in hearing.[61]

I respect Dr. Hain and his work, although, in my opinion, he is too conservative when it comes to the side effects of ototoxic drugs. He doesn't think the ototoxic side effects are as common and severe as they really are.

If you are contemplating this procedure, here are some things of which you should be aware.

First, numbers of people have a genetic variant that leaves them **very** susceptible to aminoglycoside ototoxicity—much more so than the general population. Since Gentamicin is one of the aminoglycosides, it would seem wise to be tested to see if you have the 1555A-G variant of the 12S rRNA gene (see page 123 in the 3rd edition of my book *Ototoxic Drugs Exposed* for more information on this), and if you have it, really consider whether the supposed benefit will be worth the greatly increased risk.

Second, this treatment can work great and "kill" the balance system in one ear, hopefully eliminating the severe vertigo. But what happens if later your Ménière's switches to your other ear, as it does in approximately 20% to 25% of the people with Ménière's?

With your balance system dead in one ear, you probably don't want to do the same procedure on your other ear, or you will be left without any inner ear balance function at all. Among other balance problems, this will almost certainly result in such conditions as oscillopsia (bouncing vision), ataxia (staggering gait like you were drunk), blurred vision and other problems with your eyes. If this happens to you, you will likely not drive again. You will likely find movement such as riding in a car, or even just watching action movies on your TV can make you "sick".

Third, there are no guarantees that even in low doses, the Gentamicin will not affect your hearing. Gentamicin typically damages the balance system (a good thing in this case) **more** than it damages the hearing system (a bad thing)—but this is not always the case. Are you prepared to lose some or all of your remaining hearing in that ear? It can and does happen.

If you have severe vertigo with your Ménière's, (and I can't even imagine what that must be like) and nothing else works, you may want to try this treatment. Remember, this is a treatment of "last resort"—one not to be taken lightly. What you choose is up to you. Personally, I'd never consider this until I had had my upper cervical spine (C_1 & C_2 vertebrae) checked by an upper cervical spine chiropractor and shown to be in proper alignment and yet still had intractable vertigo.

What I have said here also applies to the medium-dose and high-dose Gentamicin treatments mentioned in the following sections.

Medium-dose Gentamicin

This approach uses higher doses, of **Gentamicin**. The idea is to damage, but not totally destroy, the sensory hair cells in the vestibular system. Dr. John Shea Jr. of the Shea Clinic in Memphis, Tennessee found that by using a carefully controlled dose of **Gentamicin**, he could stop treatment as soon as there was any measurable hearing loss or vestibular damage, but before the cells in the vestibular system were completely destroyed, thus leaving the person with balance but not the vertigo.[62]

This works because the sensory cells of the balance system are typically more sensitive to damage from **Gentamicin** than are the cells of the hearing system. Thus, in theory, a carefully controlled dose can reduce vestibular function without affecting hearing. However, in practice, it is very difficult to achieve this, without also causing some degree of hearing loss.[63]

Treatment is simple. Basically, five times a day a doctor syringes the drug into the ear canal and allows it to be transported to the middle ear through a ventilating tube in the ear drum. From there it penetrates the round and oval windows into the inner ear where it influences inner ear function. The doctor stops this treatment as soon as there is any measurable hearing loss. Results from a study by Dr. Lange in Germany showed that after treatment, 88% were completely free of Ménière's symptoms, 5% had their Ménière's symptoms reduced to practically nothing, and only 7% remained unchanged.[64, 65]

A large study conducted by Dr. T. Sala of Venice, Italy, between 1974 and 1987, also using **Gentamicin**, had a similar high success rate. The vertigo attacks disappeared in 85% of the people treated for Ménière's disease. In addition, 26% found their hearing improved by at least 10 dB. For 78%, the feeling of pressure or fullness in their ears disappeared. Finally, 51% found their tinnitus completely disappeared, and the tinnitus in a further 24% was greatly reduced.[66] In a later study Dr. Sala reported greatly reduced vertigo in 86% of the people studied. Hearing improved for 19%. Hearing remained the same for 62%, and only got worse for 19%. Also, the treatment reduced or eliminated tinnitus for 62% of the people with Ménière's disease, while the feeling of fullness in the ears was partially or totally eliminated in 57% of the cases.[67]

High-dose Gentamicin

Used in high doses, intratympanic **Gentamicin** injections can totally destroy the sensory cells in the inner ear, thus stopping all hearing and balance signals to the brain. Doctors call this "chemical labyrinthectomy". This is a less invasive method than surgical labyrinthectomy, but achieves the same results. (See the sub-section on "Labyrinthectomy" in the "Surgery" section below.) Doctors may use this method when a person has intractable vertigo, and there is little hearing left to destroy.

Vestibular Implants

Researchers at various medical centers and universities around the world are working on vestibular implants to restore the balance of people with no vestibular function. Back in January, 2011, in the 3rd edition of this book, I wrote,

> There is an exciting new development in attempting to control the intractable vertigo that some people with Ménière's disease experience. That new development is a vestibular implant, currently known as the UW/Nucleus Vestibular Implant since it is being developed jointly by the University of Washington Medical Center in Seattle, WA and Cochlear Ltd. of Australia. It is essentially a cochlear implant and processor with re-engineered software and not just one, but three electrode arrays. The three electrode arrays are implanted—one electrode array in each of the three semi-circular canals in the vestibular (balance) part of the inner ear.
>
> "The idea behind this vestibular implant is to serve as a pacemaker for the inner ear," said Dr. Jay Rubinstein, the lead researcher in this project.[68] At this point, Gene Pugnetti is the first (and only) person to receive the vestibular implant in this 10-person surgical trial.[69]
>
> So far, the device has not seen active duty, but in preliminary testing with the implant, Gene explained, "They were able to turn on electrodes and give me the sensation that I was spinning—when in actuality I was sitting perfectly still".[70]
>
> Since the time doctors programmed and activated his processor, Gene hasn't had another Ménière's attack, but whenever that next attack comes and Gene activates his processor, his doctors hope his vestibular implant's signals will stop the vertigo in its tracks.

Work is continuing on developing better and better implants, but at this time (April, 2016), there are still no vestibular implants ready and approved for general use.

Surgery

For the 1 out of 10 Ménière's sufferers where all else fails to bring adequate relief, surgery is usually the last resort.[71] Surgery often does relieve the dizziness that accompanies Ménière's disease. However, it will not reduce your tinnitus or the accompanying hearing loss. There are three basic types of surgery that are available to you.

Endolymphatic Sac Shunt Surgery

This procedure attempts to drain the excess fluid out of the endolymphatic sac. This doesn't have as high a success rate as other treatments and is somewhat controversial. One of the main problems is that the shunt easily clogs up and ceases to be effective. That is probably why it initially relieves dizziness about 75% of the time, but long-term success is only about 50% or less.[72] It is not used much anymore as other treatments are more effective and less prone to problems.

Vestibular Nerve Section

If you still have hearing in the affected ear, your doctor may perform a vestibular nerve section (VNS), sometimes called a neurectomy. In this procedure, your doctor will cut the vestibular nerve that carries the balance signals to your brain. This will eliminate your vertigo about 90 percent of the time.

This surgery is not without risk, nor is it foolproof. There is roughly a 10 percent chance that you will lose all your hearing in the affected ear since the vestibular nerve and the cochlear nerve lie side by side. Thus it is easy to damage the cochlear nerve while trying to sever the vestibular nerve. Also, since the facial nerve lies in close proximity to the vestibulocochlear nerve, there is also a 2 percent chance of damage to your facial nerve during surgery. This would leave one side of your face partially paralyzed.[73] You might also end up with meningitis.[74]

There's another complicating factor. Human anatomy is not foolproof. For some reason in some people, not all the vestibular nerve fibers run in the vestibular nerve sheath like you would expect. Sometimes, some of them run in the cochlear nerve sheath. This means that just cutting the vestibular nerve does not necessarily sever all the vestibular nerve fibers. As a result, this surgery may not be successful in totally eliminating your vertigo.

Labyrinthectomy

If you have no useful hearing in the affected ear, your doctor may do a labyrinthectomy, which completely destroys your inner ear on that side. This will totally and permanently kill any hearing and balance function in that ear. You likely will be dizzy from 3 to 5 days to several weeks after the surgery, but will gradually regain your balance as your other ear takes over keeping you upright.[75] The success rate for this procedure is also about 90 percent.

With either of these two above treatments, your brain will adapt and manage without balance information coming from your operated side. As a result, you will be able to resume normal activity.

The down side to these two above treatments is that since you must now rely on the balance system in your other ear, if your Ménière's should later develop in the other side, your vertigo will often be much worse than if you hadn't undergone either of these treatments.

Chapter 5 Endnotes

1 Upper Cervical Chiropractic, 2015.
2 Burcon, ~2011.
3 Burcon, 2015c.
4 Buchanan, 2015d.
5 Upper Cervical Chiropractic, 2015.
6 Buchanan, 2015d.
7 Burcon, 2015c.
8 Burcon, 2015c.
9 Burcon, 2015c.
10 Upper Cervical Chiropractic, 2015.
11 Buchanan, 2015b.
12 Blair Upper Cervical Chiropractic Society, Inc., 2014.
13 Buchanan, 2015e.
14 Buchanan, 2015c.
15 Salt, 1998d. p. 1.
16 Salt, 2005. p. 6.
17 Hydrops and Ménière's Diet Suggestions, 1996. p. 1.
18 Ménière's Disease, 1997. p. 3.
19 Gates, 2004. p. 719.
20 Hain, 2011a. p. 9.
21 Salt, 1998c. p. 2.
22 Hazell, 1982.
23 Ménière's Disease, 1997. p. 4.
24 Endolymphatic Hydrops, 1996.
25 Hain, 2009c. p. 2.
26 Hydrops and Ménière's Diet Suggestions, 1996.

27 Ménière's Disease, 1997. p. 3.
28 Rezen, 1985. p. 90.
29 Ménière's Disease, 1997. pp. 3-4.
30 Auto Immune Disease: New Discoveries for Less Pain & Less Meds for Auto Immune Diseases, 2011. pp. 1-2.
31 Hyman, 2010. p. 2.
32 Is There a Cure for Ménière's Disease? 2011. pp. 1-2.
33 Hyman, 2010. p2.
34 Hyman, 2010. p. 3.
35 Hyman, 2010. p. 3.
36 Gibson, 2003. p. 2.
37 Bjorne, 2003. p. 1
38 Hain, 2010d. p. 3.
39 Hain, 2011a, p. 7.
40 Salt, 1998c. pp. 1-2.
41 Hain, 2011a. p. 6.
42 Hain, 2010a. pp. 2-3.
43 Shea, 1996. pp. 353-358.
44 Garduno-Anaya, 2005. p. 1.
45 Hain, 2011a. p. 6.
46 Miller, 1998. p. 2.
47 Ménière's Disease, 1997. p. 4.
48 Delving Into The Many Mysteries Of Ménière's Disease, 1991. pp. 2 & 9.
49 Controlling Ménière's Disease Brightens A Life, 1991. p. 3.
50 Gates, 2002. p. 1491.
51 Ménière's Disease and the Meniett Low-Pressure Pulse Generator, 2002. p. 4.
52 Odkvist, 2000. p. 101.
53 Hain, 2011b. pp. 2-3.
54 Gates, 2002. p. 1490.
55 Gates, 2006. p.1.
56 Gates, 2004. p. 721.
57 Suitable Patients, 2006. p. 1.
58 Ménière's Disease and the Meniett Low-Pressure Pulse Generator, 2002. p. 24.
59 van der Laan, Franz. 2005. p. 1.
60 Pyykko, I. 1994. pp. 162-167.
61 Hain, 2010b. pp. 1-2.
62 Shea, 1994. pp. 317-324.
63 Salt, 1998c. p. 6.
64 Lange, 1989. pp. 269-270.
65 Lange, 1995. pp. 720-723.
66 Sala, 1988. pp. 293-296.
67 Sala, 1997. pp. 239-246.
68 UW Ménière's implant passes first test, 2010. p. 1.
69 First Device Implanted to Treat Balance Disorder, 2010. p. 1.
70 UW Ménière's implant passes first test, 2010. p. 1.
71 Delving Into The Many Mysteries Of Ménière's Disease, 1991. p. 9.
72 Ménière's Disease, 1997. p. 5.
73 Vernick, 1993. pp. 174-175.
74 Ménière's Disease, 1997. p. 5.
75 Ménière's Disease, 1997. p. 6.

Chapter 6

Tips for Living with Ménière's Disease

Ménière's attacks are unpredictable. Furthermore, these attacks are not high on the list of "fun things" you want to experience again. In fact, after you've had a severe attack of vertigo, you fervently hope that another attack will never happen in the future.

Since Ménière's attacks are unpredictable, when you leave home, you never know whether you might experience another Ménière's attack while you are out. This can lead to anxiety, and, in extreme cases, a person becomes afraid to leave home.

In fact, the fear of another Ménière's attack can demoralize you more than the actual attack. You are always anxious because you constantly fear another attack at the most inopportune time. You may be afraid to continue activities such as driving a car or operating machinery. You may feel safer cloistered in your own home, rather than risking having an attack while out with friends or while attending an event.[1]

Be assured, you need to live, work and drive as normal between episodes. Although Ménière's attacks come on unexpectedly, you usually have enough warning to allow you to stop driving, to put down a dangerous instrument or to get off a ladder,[2] although if you are prone to "drop attacks", you won't have any warning whatsoever.

One of the best practical steps you can take to help alleviate extreme anxiety is to plan ahead of time the steps you will need to take if a Ménière's attack should occur unexpectedly. Be sure to include an "escape route" in your plan so you will have a safe place nearby where you can go to recover from a

Ménière's attack. With a good plan in place, you will find that you are much less anxious than you would be otherwise.

It can be scary if you are out driving and a Ménière's attack comes on, but take heart, if you have a good plan, you typically will be able to cope. Here's how "Carl" does it. He explained:

> I occasionally experienced vertigo attacks while driving. At first, they came on slowly and I could feel something was not right. Later, they came on abruptly with a spinning sensation starting without any warning. Many times I would start out on an errand in the car and turn back after a block or so because I realized that I was about to get vertigo.
>
> I dealt with these in a couple of ways. First, I always had in mind an "escape route". I'd keep in mind some place I could go to let the vertigo wear off. It might be a place to park the car for a few hours, or the house of a friend or relative along my route.
>
> I also would tell myself that it is only an illusion. The car is not spinning, and I am not spinning. Everything is moving along in a normal way. As I thought this, I'd find a way to pull over to the side of the road or to get off the freeway.
>
> More than once, I realized a vertigo attack was imminent and simply did not go where I wanted to. It might mean that I stayed home, or that I remained at work till I began feeling better. But often those attacks lasted 8 to 24 hours, so remaining at work wasn't a good option. In that case, I'd call someone to see if they could drive me home.
>
> After my second ear became afflicted, the attacks changed so that they came on like lightening. I'd be standing one moment and then suddenly be grabbing for anything to keep from falling the next minute. It became too unpredictable to drive. I was even hesitant to walk to the mail box 100 feet up the street, not knowing if I'd make it back to the house. I never went anywhere without knowing of an "escape route" or place I could go to crash.

"Candice" also has had vertigo attacks while driving. She explained:

> I have only had two drop attacks while driving, and those were probably some of the scariest moments of my life. There was nothing I could do but pull over—it felt like I was slowing down horribly and zig-zagging in traffic.

"Colleen" once got waylaid by a Ménière's attack while driving. She related:

> All of a sudden the road was not straight, and it was moving in ways that roads shouldn't move. I pulled over to the side of the road and called my daughter-in-law. I was vomiting by the side of the road until she got to me.
>
> Since then, I have been having problems—especially when driving. The sun during the day will start it, or the headlights of oncoming cars. I am not driving much now because I have no idea when I am going to have an attack.

Your Ménière's may affect your sensation of acceleration and deceleration. As Alan explained,

> I don't feel acceleration unless it is strong. The fact I can't detect subtle changes in acceleration causes me to avoid driving in snow and ice. I just don't trust my ability to discern the subtle changes you can get driving in slippery conditions.
>
> Furthermore, if my wife is driving, I may feel as if she's not going to stop at an intersection because I've not felt the gradual slowing of the car. However, if I'm pressed back in my seat, as on an airliner taking off, I am aware of the acceleration.

Tracy has similar problems. She related,

> I'm feeling a bit sheepish because recently I've really been fussing at my husband for speeding towards cars in front of us that have the brake lights on. I mean **really** fussing! He swears he slowing down, but I am convinced he is accelerating toward them. I'm afraid I may have to apologize to him...just this once!

You don't have to like your Ménière's disease and resulting vertigo. (Who does?) Alan explained:

> If I had a choice between regaining my hearing or regaining normal balance, I'd take balance in a heartbeat. Lack of inner ear balance limits a lot of things you can do. It makes it hard to walk in poor lighting or darkness; it makes walking in a crowd almost impossible; it keeps me from driving on the freeway or at night; it causes oscillopsia (bouncing vision); and it generally impedes me from doing things I used to really enjoy like riding a bicycle or skiing.

However, you don't have to let Ménière's disease take over your whole life and prevent you from doing some of the things you want to do. You may have to do them differently, but they may still be doable. Alan recounted:

> One thing pleasantly surprised me. About 12 years ago, we started going to Hawaii each year. At that time, a physical therapist I was working with cautioned me about swimming in the ocean as she was concerned I'd become disoriented. I got there, looked at the pristine waters of the bay and said, "To heck with it, I'm going in!" I'd been a lifeguard and swimming instructor for many years, and I am very at home in the water.
>
> To my surprise, when I got my snorkel gear on and out in the bay, I felt **normal** for the first time in years. I think it was because of the lack of the importance of gravity, and not having to balance myself to avoid falling. Even in fairly rough water, I feel fine.

Alan added:

> One advantage of not having any inner ear balance—no motion sickness. We regularly fly a little island hopper between Oahu and Maui—a rough ride many times—but I can just sit back and smile as others onboard reach for the barf bags!

Following are some lifestyle hints which fellow Ménière's sufferers have found helpful. Try them and see what works for you.

- As mentioned previously, avoid whatever triggers your Ménière's attacks as much as you can.
- Do not over-exert yourself.
- Avoid undue stress at all times. Ménière's attacks frequently hit during (or immediately following) times of severe stress or fatigue.[3] Interestingly enough, many Ménière's sufferers are "Type A" personalities—easily stressed, self-motivated and over-achievers.[4] If this is you, learn to relax and not get so uptight over everything. If your Ménière's attacks are related to stress, you need to learn how to get your stress under control; or to avoid stressful situations as much as possible. Doing so can reduce the incidence and the severity of your Ménière's attacks.
- Get out of bed slowly. It helps to sit on the edge of the bed for a minute before standing up.
- Turn your head slowly because this can cause disequilibrium or vertigo. This also includes when looking from side to side, or looking over your shoulder. As Leigh explained, "Fast movements to the side make me spin." Carol related, "In order to see something behind me, I must first stop, and then slowly turn around."

John reported,

> I had problems with head movement causing dizziness pretty bad when I was initially diagnosed with Ménière's, but it seems less so now that my eyes seem to have taken over much of the balance effort. I initially had problems riding my bicycle (which I love), but now I'm pretty good if I don't look around too much while riding.

One man explained,

> Just turning my head sharply while backing up my car caused a Ménière's attack. Even now, I have to move my head gingerly, or I risk feelings of disequilibrium.

- If you have severe problems with your balance when you are out walking or hiking, use a walker, cane, hiking stick or umbrella to steady yourself.
- When riding in a car or on a bus, try to sit on the curb (passenger) side because the traffic whizzing past on the other side may affect you, especially at night as the lights flash past. If riding in a vehicle bothers you, take this one step further and sit in the back seat of a car or near the rear of a bus. You may find it really helps if you shut your eyes.
- Avoid visual stimuli that trigger your Ménière's attacks. Many people with Ménière's report that certain things, especially parallel vertical lines, will trigger their dizziness and other symptoms. Some of these visual stimuli include streets lined with trees or telephone poles, visually "busy" supermarket aisles and even some motion pictures.[5]
- A group of people with severely-damaged vestibular systems due to Ménière's disease shared the below list of visual triggers that often cause them grief. These are the situations you want to avoid if possible. This list of visual triggers includes:
  - Watching a big screen TV or going to movie theaters
  - Looking up/down suddenly
  - Walking down a visually-busy aisle in a store
  - Driving on a "cloverleaf" highway ramp
  - Walking beside flowing water such as a river (as opposed to walking beside a lake)

    - Cars rushing by as you walk down a road
    - Walking on a track with joggers zipping by
    - Cars speeding in the opposite direction as you are driving on a narrow road
    - Walking in the dark, or on a dimly lit path
    - Looking back in response to a call
    - Zipping past street lights while riding in a motor vehicle
    - Walking in a crowd
    - Sailing in a small boat vs. in a large ship
    - Moving lights, especially in a disco, and moving lights at night when driving
    - Bicycles zipping by
    - Walking up or down steps
    - Walking in a steeply sloped theater or arena, or on any incline

- Be careful of walking on inclines. That can mess up your sense of balance. As Alan explains,

> I have balance difficulties in situations such as a theater or stadium with sloping floors. One of the hardest places for me is the ramp leading onto an airliner because of a peculiar optical illusion that is built into those ramps.

Tracy has similar problems with inclines. She found she now has trouble walking in a restaurant where her family often dines. She discovered that "what was tripping me up was that there was a very slight incline as you enter".

- Walk in the middle of the sidewalk. That way if you lurch and stagger during an attack, you will not crash into a store window, or lurch off the sidewalk into the road.

- When sitting down, try to sit in a chair with arms or sit near something you can hold.

- Before crossing a road, stand still at the curb, slowly turn your head from side to side to see if any traffic is coming, then walk firmly straight ahead.

- When getting a bit flustered, stand still, take a couple of deep breaths and "gather yourself together".[6]

- Join a Ménière's self-help support group and learn as many tips as you can from fellow Ménière's sufferers, and from the literature they provide. (See "Sources of Help" for contact information.)

- Explain to your family and friends what might happen when you have a Ménière's attack and what you want them to do. Then, if you have an attack when they are present, they will understand what is happening. They will know what to do and will not be frightened.

- If you have a bad attack, in order to minimize its effects, immediately lie down on a firm surface. Stay as motionless as possible. Keep your eyes open and fixed on a stationary object some distance away. Do not drink anything because you may vomit. Remain like this until the room stops spinning, then get up **very slowly**. After such an episode you will likely be very tired and will need to sleep for several hours.[7]

- If your balance system has been damaged, you will find it better (easier) to walk on firm, even surfaces, rather than on loose or uneven surfaces such as sand, snow, a rough path, etc. Furthermore, wear firm walking shoes rather than sandals or loose shoes.

- Also, if your balance system has been damaged, you will rely much more on your eyes. Thus you will find it much more difficult to keep your balance when it is dark or the light is poor. For example, Alan explained,

  > When I go camping, I have to get everything done by the time it becomes dark. As the light fades, so does my ability to balance, and when it's dark, and the ground is uneven and lit only by a flickering fire or flashlight, I can barely get around.

- If you are plagued with imbalance problems between your Ménière's attacks, you may find it worthwhile to have vestibular therapy. Vestibular therapy works at retraining your brain to better process your (now-faulty) balance information, to develop skills to compensate for impaired balance, and to better cope with vertigo attacks.[8] Vestibular rehabilitation exercises are a form of physical therapy. One of the secrets to successful therapy is to make a concerted effort to keep moving and exercising in spite of your feelings of dizziness and imbalance. The good news is that your balance will improve over the months as you constantly exercise your vestibular system.

Chapter 6 Endnotes

1 Adey, 1989.
2 Engel, 1993. pp. 161-162.
3 Ménière's Disease, 1997. p. 4.
4 Salt, 1998d. p. 3.
5 Hines, 1997. p 4.
6 Nobbs. p. 32.
7 Ménière's Disease, 1996.
8 Gibson, 2003. p. 2.

Chapter 7

Sources of Help for Ménière's Disease

Good Sources of Information for People with Ménière's Disease

Center for Hearing Loss Help
Internet: http://hearinglosshelp.com/blog/topic/ear-problems/menieres-disease/

Currently there are 10 articles on Ménière's disease by the author of this book. In addition, there are about 900 articles related to various aspects of hearing loss, tinnitus, coping strategies, assistive devices, etc.

Burcon Chiropractic Ménière's Research Institute
Internet: http://www.burconchiropractic.com/page/2879

This is Dr. Burcon's website showing how Ménière's disease is caused by C_1 and C_2 vertebrae out of alignment. It includes 5 hours of YouTube "Health Talks" and other information.

Note: While the below websites are good sources of information on Ménière's disease, all of them miss the boat as they do not talk about the underlying cause of Ménière's disease—namely C_1 and C_2 vertebrae out of alignment. So read their information with this in mind.

Ménière's Disease
Internet: http://www.dizziness-and-balance.com/disorders/menieres/menieres.html

This is an excellent up-to-date source of authoritative information on Ménière's disease by Dr. Timothy Hain.

Menieres-Help.Com
Internet: http://www.menieres-help.com/index.php

This website gives you hope. It features people who have had Ménière's disease and beaten it and now live symptom-free by using top-quality dietary supplements.

Ménière's Disease Information Center
Internet: http://www.menieresinfo.com/

This is an up-to-date comprehensive on-line resource for information about Ménière's disease.

Good Sources of Support for People with Ménière's Disease

Vestibular Disorders Association (VEDA)
Box 13305
Portland, OR 97213
Voice 1-800-837-8428
FAX 1-503-229-8064
Internet: www.vestibular.org

VEDA provides information and support to people suffering from inner-ear balance disorders. They have a lot of information on-line at their web page including an excellent list of support groups in Canada and the USA.

SayWhat Club (SWC) Ménière's List
Internet: http://www.saywhatclub.com

If you have Ménière's disease and want on-line support and friendship, consider joining the SayWhatClub's Ménière's list.

To join the SayWhatClub (SWC), click on http://www.saywhatclub.com/, then click on the "Join Us" button. There it explains about the SWC, and how you can join. When you contact the SWC, a person from the SayWhatClub's hospitality committee will contact you and guide you through the process. Tell them you want to join the Ménière's list. You will be welcome!

Literature Cited

> **Obsolete URLs**
>
> **Note**: Many of the URLs from which information was cited no longer exist. Obsolete URLs (as of April, 2016) are shown in square brackets. The information obtained from now obsolete links may still exist on the Internet at another URL if you want to try and track down that particular information.

Adey, Muriel. 1989. Letter re Ménière's Disease. In: *CHHA Communiqué*. Vol. 6. No. 4. 1989.

Auto Immune Disease: New Discoveries for Less Pain & Less Meds for Auto Immune Diseases. 2011. http://www.healthdiscoveries.net/auto-immune-disease.html.

Bauman, Neil. 2011. Protect Your Balance System—Or Else. http://hearinglosshelp.com/blog/protect-your-balance-system-or-else/.

Blair Upper Cervical Chiropractic Society, Inc. 2014. Repairing the Body and Health Outcomes. http://www.blairchiropractic.com/repairing-the-body-and-health-outcomes.

Bjorne, A. 2003. Symptom Relief After Treatment of Temporomandibular and Cervical Spine Disorders in Patients with Ménière's Disease: A Three-year Follow-up. Cranio. 2003 Jan; 21(1): 50-60. Abstract in PubMed. http://www.ncbi.nlm.nih.gov/pubmed/12555932?dopt=Abstract.

Buchanan, Greg. 2015a. Blair Upper Cervical—Dr. William G. Blair. http://www.upcspine.com/tech3.htm.

Buchanan, Greg. 2015b. My Findings. http://www.upcspine.com/intro.htm.

Buchanan, Greg. 2015c. Conditions That Respond. http://www.upcspine.com/respond.htm.

Buchanan, Greg. 2015d. Introduction to Upper Cervical Techniques. http://www.upcspine.com/approach1.htm.

Buchanan, Greg. 2015e. Sign/Symptom Checklist. http://www.upcspine.com/self.htm.

Burcon, Michael. 2005. Upper Cervical Protocol for Thirty Ménière's Patients. [http://www.burconchiropractic.com/images/files/b626_file5_545.pdf].

Burcon, Michael. 2010. Upper Cervical Protocol & Results for 300 Ménière's Patients. Sixth International Symposium on Ménière's Disease. Kyoto, Japan. [http://www.burconchiropractic.com/g5-bin/client.cgi?G5button=626&subcategoryID=1259].

Burcon, Michael. ~2011. Cervical Specific Protocol & Results for 300 Ménière's Patients. Presented at the New Zealand College of Chiropractic, Upper Cervical Conference. [http://www.burconchiropractic.com/g5-bin/client.cgi?G5button=626&subcategoryID=2525].

Burcon, Michael. 2015a. Winter Newsletter. [http://www.burconchiropractic.com/g5-bin/client.cgi?G5button=626&subcategoryID=2569].

Burcon, Michael. 2015b. Burcon Chiropractic. http://www.burconchiropractic.com.

Burcon, Michael. 2015c. Personal communication.

Controlling Ménière's Disease Brightens a Life. 1991. In: *Oto Review*. House Ear Institute. Affiliated with the University of Southern California. Spring, 1991.

Delving into the Many Mysteries of Ménière's Disease. 1991. In: *Oto Review*. House Ear Institute. Affiliated with the University of Southern California. Spring, 1991.

Endolymphatic Hydrops. 1996. The Vestibular Disorders Association (VEDA). [http://www.teleport.com/~veda].

Engel, June. 1993. The Complete Canadian Health Guide. University of Toronto, Faculty of Medicine. Key Porter Books, Toronto, Ontario.

First Device Implanted to Treat Balance Disorder, Nov. 18, 2010. Hearing Review. [http://www.hearingreview.com/insider/2010-11-18_05.asp].

Garduno-Anaya, M. A., et. al. 2005. Dexamethasone Inner Ear Perfusion by Intratympanic Injection in Unilateral Ménière's Disease: a Two-year Prospective, Placebo-Controlled, Double-Blind, Randomized Trial. Otolaryngol Head Neck Surg. 2005 Aug; 133(2): 285-94. http://www.ncbi.nlm.nih.gov/pubmed/16087029?dopt=Abstract.

Gates, G. A. & J. Douglas Green. 2002. Intermittent Pressure Therapy of Intractable Ménière's Disease Using the Meniett Device: A Preliminary Report. Laryngoscope 112: August 2002.

Gates, G. A., et. al. 2004. The Effects of Transtympanic Micropressure Treatment in People with Unilateral Ménière's Disease. Arch Otolaryngol Head Neck Surg. Vol 130, June 2004. pp. 718-725.

Gates, G. A., et. al. 2006. Meniett Clinical Trial: Long-Term Follow-Up. In: Arch Otolaryngol Head Neck Surg. 2006 Dec; 132(12): 1311-6.

Gibson, Bill. 2003. Ménière's Disease. http://www.healthinsite.gov.au/expert/Meniere_s_Disease.

Hain, Timothy. 2009a. Epidemiology of Ménière's Disease. http://www.dizziness-and-balance.com/disorders/menieres/men_epi.html.

Hain, Timothy. 2009b. Drop Attacks. http://www.dizziness-and-balance.com/disorders/central/drop.html.

Hain, Timothy. 2009c. Hydrops and Hydrops Diet. http://www.dizziness-and-balance.com/disorders/menieres/hydrops.html.

Hain, Timothy. 2010a. Last Resort Treatments of Severe Ménière's Disease. http://www.dizziness-and-balance.com/disorders/menieres/menieres%20last%20resort.html.

Hain, Timothy. 2010b. Intratympanic/Transtympanic Gentamicin Treatment for Ménière's Disease. http://www.dizziness-and-balance.com/treatment/ttg.html.

Hain, Timothy. 2010c. Autoimmune Inner Ear Disease (AIED). http://www.dizziness-and-balance.com/disorders/autoimmune/aied.html.

Hain, Timothy. 2010d. Drug Treatment of Vertigo. http://www.dizziness-and-balance.com/treatment/drug/drugrx.html.

Hain, Timothy. 2011a. Ménière's Disease. http://www.dizziness-and-balance.com/disorders/menieres/menieres.html.

Hain, Timothy. 2011b. Ménière's Disease—Treatments That May Be Placebos. http://www.dizziness-and-balance.com/disorders/menieres/menieres_placebo.htm.

Hazell, J. W. P. 1982. Ménière's Disease. In: British Tinnitus Association Newsletter. Newsletter 16, April, 1982.

Heselsweet, Geraldine. 1999. Success Story. [http://www.burconchiropractic.com/g5-bin/client.cgi?G5button=626&articleID=935].

Hines, Ray. 1997. Ménière's Org Information Center. [http://www.menieres.org/moic.htm].

Hogan, Kevin. 1998. Tinnitus: Turning the Volume Down. Proven Strategies for Turning the Noise Down in Your Head. Network 3000 Publishing Co. Eagan. MN 55123.

Hydrops and Ménière's Diet Suggestions, 1996. The Vestibular Disorders Association (VEDA). [http://www.teleport.com/~veda].

Hyman, Mark. 2010. Glutathione: The Mother of All Antioxidants. http://www.huffingtonpost.com/dr-mark-hyman/glutathione-the-mother-of_b_530494.html.

Is There a Cure for Ménière's Disease? 2011. http://www.glutathionediseasecure.com/cure-for-menieres-disease.html.

Lange, G. 1989. Gentamicin and Other Ototoxic Antibiotics for the Transtympanic Treatment of Ménière's Disease. In: *Archives of Oto-Rhino-Laryngology/Head and Neck Surgery.* 246 (5) pp. 269-270.

Lange, G. 1995. 27 Years Experiences with Transtympanic Aminoglycoside Treatment of Ménière's Disease. In: *Laryngorhinootologie* 1995 Dec; 74(12): pp. 720-723.

Lermoyez Syndrome. 2011. The Free Dictionary. http://medical-dictionary.thefreedictionary.com/Lermoyez+syndrome.

Ménière's Disease. 1996. The Vestibular Disorders Association (VEDA). [http://www.teleport.com/~veda].

Ménière's Disease. 1997. Answers to Common Otolaryngology Health Care Questions. Department of Otolaryngology—Head and Neck Surgery. University of Washington School of Medicine. [http://weber.u.washington.edu/~otoweb/meniere.html].

Ménière's Disease. 2010. Vestibular Disorders Association. https://vestibular.org/menieres-disease.

Ménière's Disease and the Meniett Low-Pressure Pulse Generator. 2002. Medtronic Xomed. Jacksonville, FL 32216.

Miller, Larry. 1998. The Chronology of a Ménière's Disease Victim's Suffering and Success. [http://www.vcnet.com/lmiller/MyStory.html].

Nobbs, Marie. The Ménière's Group. In: *C.H.I.P. Background Information For Speechreading Instructors.* Extracted from various issues of the British publication, *Catchword.*

Odkvist, L. M., et. al. 2000. Effects of Middle Ear Pressure Changes on Clinical Symptoms in Patients with Ménière's Disease—a Clinical Multicentre Placebo-Controlled Study. Acta Otolaryngol 2000; Suppl 543: 99-101.

Pyykko, I. 1994. Intratympanic Gentamicin in Bilateral Ménière's Disease. In: *Archives of Oto-Rhino-Laryngology/Head and Neck Surgery.* 110 (2) pp. 162-167.

Rezen, Susan & Carl Hausman. 1985. Coping with Hearing Loss: A Guide for Adults and Their Families. Dembner Books, New York, N.Y.

Sala, T. 1988. Transtympanic Administration of Aminoglycosides in Patients with Ménière's Disease. In: *Archives of Oto-Rhino-Laryngology/Head and Neck Surgery.* 245 (5) pp. 293-296.

Sala, T. 1997. Transtympanic Gentamicin in the Treatment of Ménière's Disease. In: *Auris Nasus Larynx.* Jul. 24(3) pp. 239-246.

Salt, Alec N. 1998a. Symptoms and Incidence of Ménière's Disease. [http://oto.wustl.edu/men/mn1.htm].

Salt, Alec N. 1998b. Origins and Causes of Ménière's Disease. [http://oto.wustl.edu/men/mn5.htm].

Salt, Alec N. 1998c. Compilation of Treatments for Ménière's Disease. [http://oto.wustl.edu/men/mn7.htm].

Salt, Alec N. 1998d. Frequently Asked Questions. [http://oto.wustl.edu/men/mn3.htm].

Salt, Alec N. 1998e. Cochlear Fluids Composition. [http://oto.wustl.edu/cochlea/intro3.htm].

Salt, Alec N. 1998f. Endolymphatic Hydrops. [http://oto.wustl.edu/cochlea/intro4.htm].

Salt, Alec N. 1998g. Measurement of Endolymph Flow Rate. [http://oto.wustl.edu/cochlea/res1.htm].

Salt, Alec N. 2005. Frequently Asked Questions (FAQ). [http://oto2.wustl.edu/men/mnfaq.htm#Q12label].

Shea, John J. Jr. 1993. Classification of Ménière's Disease. In: *American Journal of Otology*. 14 (3). pp. 224-229. May, 1993.

Shea, John J. Jr. 1994. Streptomycin Perfusion of the Labyrinth Through the Round Window Plus Intravenous Streptomycin. In: *Otolaryngologic Clinics of North America*. 27(2): 317-324. April, 1994.

Shea, John J. Jr. 1996. Dexamethasone Perfusion of the Labyrinth Plus Intravenous Dexamethasone for Ménière's Disease. In: *Otolaryngologic Clinics of North America*. 29(2): 353-358. April, 1996.

Suitable Patients. 2006. [www.meniett.com/device_suitable_patients.html].

Tyrrell, J. S., et. al. Prevalence, Associated Factors, and Comorbid Conditions for Ménière's Disease. Ear and Hearing (April 2014). Reported in: Tinnitus Today. Summer, 2014.

Upper Cervical Chiropractic. 2015. FAQ. http://www.upper-cervical.com/html/faq.html.

UW Ménière's Implant Passes First Test. Nov. 19, 2010. King 5 HealthLink. [http://www.king5.com/health/Menieres-implant-passes-first-test-109301209.html].

van der Laan, Franz. 2005. P-100 in the Treatment of Ménière's Disease: a Clinical Study. In: Int. Tinnitus J. 2005: 11(2): 146-9. http://www.ncbi.nlm.nih.gov/pubmed/16639914?dopt=Abstract.

Vernick, David M. & Constance Grzelka. 1993. The Hearing Loss Handbook. Consumer Reports Books. Yonkers, N.Y.

Wikipedia. 2011. Marcel Lermoyez. http://en.wikipedia.org/wiki/Marcel_Lermoyez.

Good Books on Hearing Loss

Integrity First Books in the series:

Everything You Wanted to Know About Your Hearing Loss But Were Afraid to Ask (Because You Knew You Wouldn't Hear the Answers Anyway!)

by Neil G. Bauman, Ph.D.

If you have enjoyed this book and would like to learn more about hearing loss and how you can successfully live with it, you may be interested in some helpful books by Dr. Neil. Each book is packed with the things you need to know in order to thrive in spite of your various hearing loss issues. The direct link to the following books is at http://hearinglosshelp.com/shop/category/books/.

Ototoxic Drugs Exposed—The Shocking Truth About Prescription Drugs, Medications, Chemicals and Herbals That Can (and Do) Damage Our Ears
($52.45; eBook $39.95)

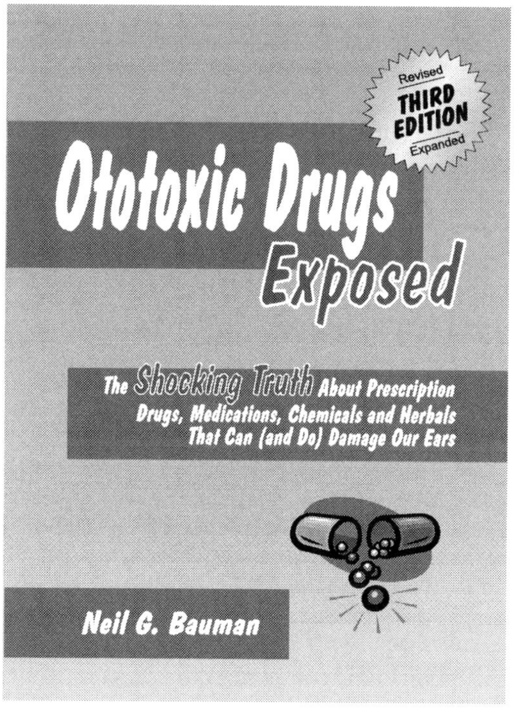

This book, now in its third edition, reveals the shocking truth that many prescription drugs can damage your ears. Some drugs slowly and insidiously rob you of your hearing, cause your ears to ring or destroy your balance. Other drugs can smash your ears in one fell swoop, leaving you with profound, permanent hearing loss and bringing traumatic change into your life. Learn how to protect your ears from the ravages of ototoxic drugs and chemicals. Describes the specific ototoxic effects of 877 drugs, 35 herbals and 148 chemicals (798 pages).

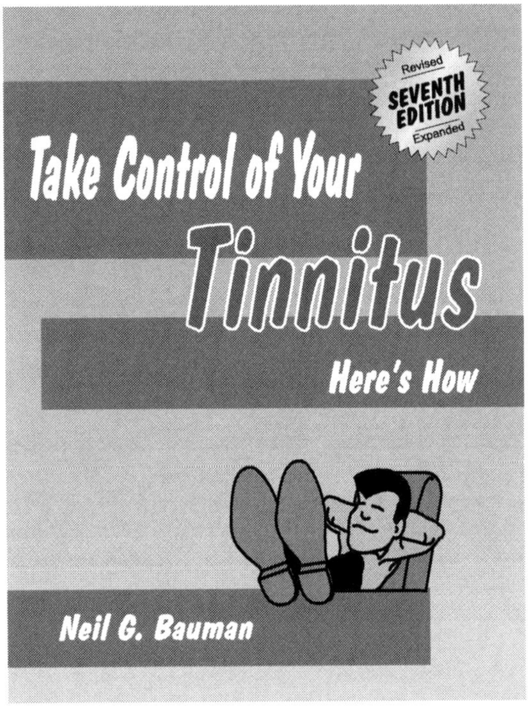

Take Control of Your Tinnitus—Here's How ($29.95; eBook $22.99)

If your ears ring, buzz, chirp, hiss, click or roar, you know just how annoying tinnitus can be. The good news is that you do not have to put up with this racket for the rest of your life. You can take control of your tinnitus. Recent studies show that a lot of what we thought we knew about tinnitus is not true at all. Exciting new research reveals a number of things that you can do to eliminate or greatly reduce the severity of your tinnitus so that it no longer bothers you. This totally-revised, up-to-date and expanded 7th edition contains the very latest in tinnitus research and treatment. In this book you will learn what tinnitus is, what causes tinnitus and things you can do to take control of your tinnitus (356 pages).

Phantom Voices, Ethereal Music & Other Spooky Sounds ($22.49; eBook $16.99)

When you realize you are hearing phantom sounds, you immediately think that something has gone dreadfully wrong "upstairs"—that you are going crazy. Because of this, few people openly talk about the strange phantom voices, music, singing and other spooky sounds they hear. This book, the first of its kind in the world, lifts the veil on "Musical Ear syndrome" and reveals numerous first-hand accounts of the many strange phantom sounds people experience. Not only that, it explains what causes these phantom sounds, and more importantly, what you can do to eliminate them, or at least, bring them under control (178 pages).

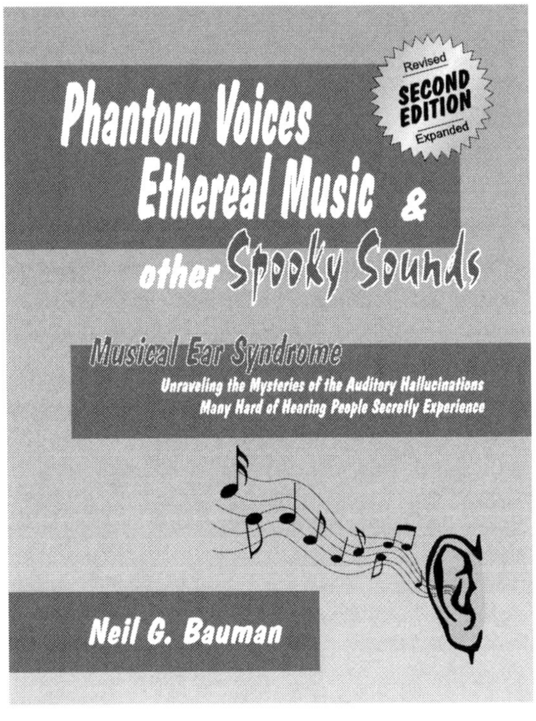

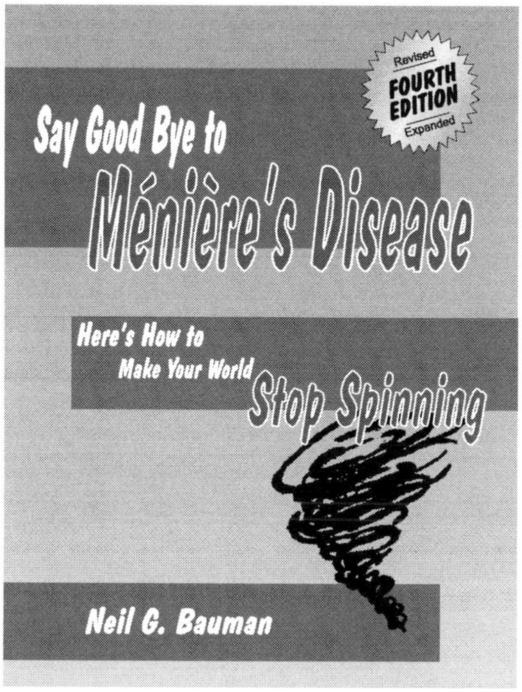

Say Good Bye to Ménière's Disease—Here's How to Make Your World Stop Spinning ($21.95; eBook $16.49)

Ménière's disease is one of the more baffling and incapacitating conditions a person can experience. If you suffer from your world spinning, have a fluctuating hearing loss, tinnitus and a feeling of fullness in your ears, this book is for you. It details what Ménière's disease is like; explains the recent breakthrough into the underlying cause of Ménière's; and shows you how, at last, you can be free from the ravages of this debilitating condition. Each page is packed with practical information to help you successfully conquer your Meniere's disease. Join the hundreds and hundreds of people whose worlds have now stopped spinning (128 pages).

Keys to Successfully Living with Your Hearing Loss ($19.97; eBook $15.49)

Do you know: a) the critical missing element to successfully living with your hearing loss? b) that the No. 1 coping strategy hard of hearing people instinctively use is wrong, wrong, wrong? c) what the single most effective hearing loss coping strategy is? d) how you can turn your hearing aids into awesome hearing devices? This book addresses the surprising answers to these and other critical questions. Applying them to your life will put you well on the road to successfully living with your hearing loss (84 pages).

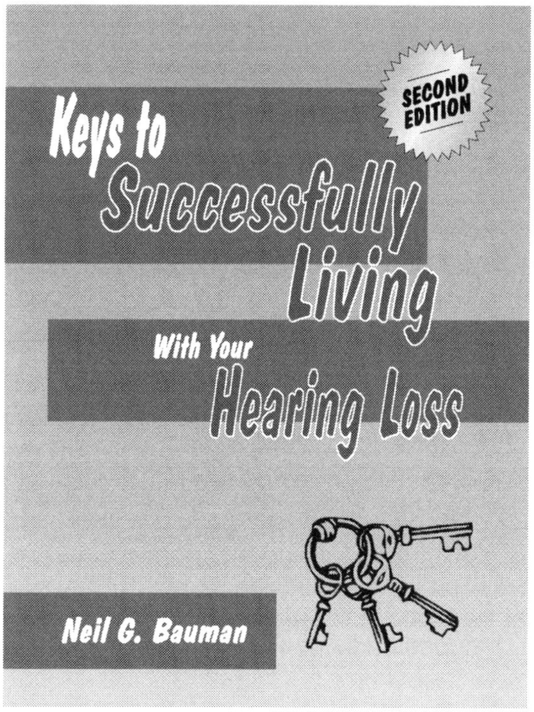

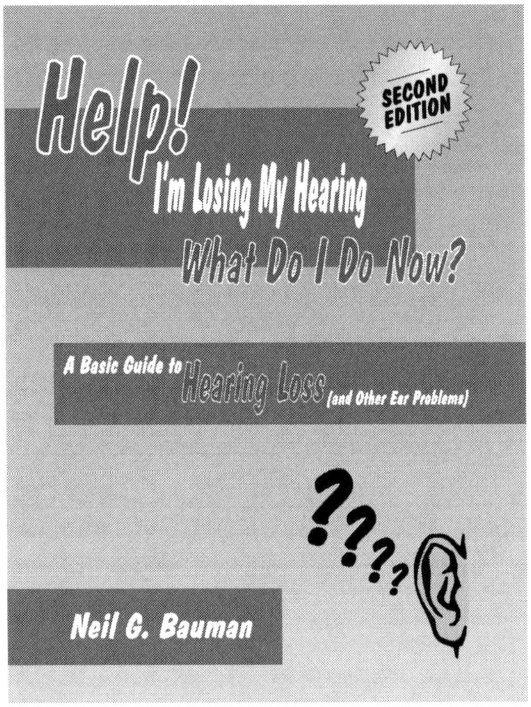

Help! I'm Losing My Hearing—What Do I Do Now? ($18.95; eBook $14.49)

Losing your hearing can flip your world upside down and leave your mind in a turmoil. You may be full of fears, wondering how you will be able to live the rest of your life as a hard of hearing person. You don't know where to turn. You lament, "What do I do now?" Set your mind at rest. This easy to read book, written by a fellow hard of hearing person, is packed with the information and resources you need to successfully deal with your hearing loss and other ear conditions (116 pages).

Grieving for Your Hearing Loss—The Rocky Road from Denial to Acceptance ($12.95; eBook $9.95)

When you lose your hearing you need to grieve. This is not optional—but critical to your continued mental and physical health. This book leads you through the process of dealing with the grief and pain you experience as a result of your hearing loss. It explains what you are going through each step of the way. It gives you hope when you are in the depths of despair and depression. It shows you how you can lead a happy vibrant life again in spite of your hearing loss. This book has helped many (56 pages).

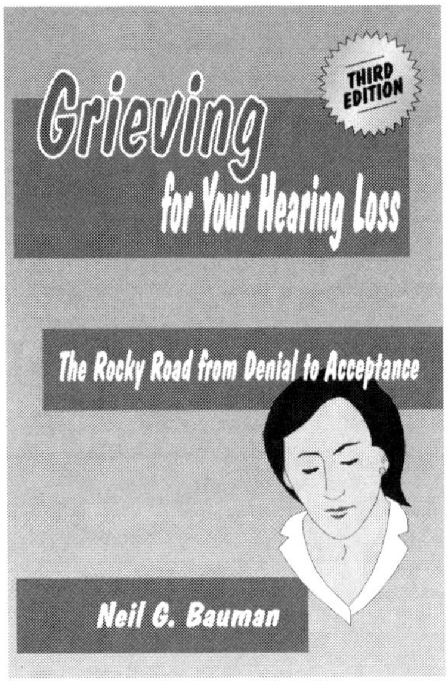

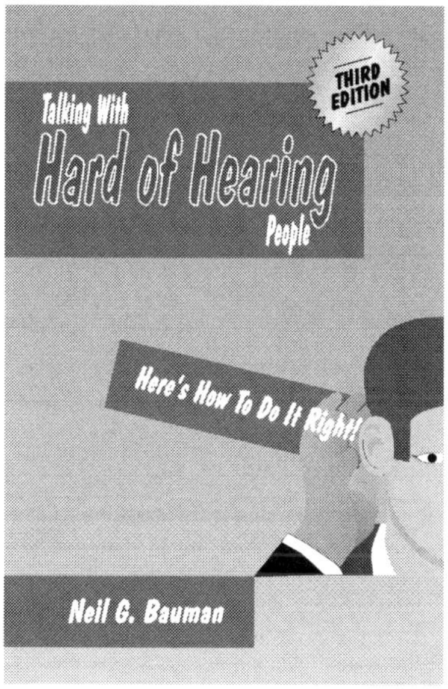

Talking with Hard of Hearing People—Here's How to Do It Right! ($9.95; eBook $7.95)

Talking is important to all of us. When communication breaks down, we all suffer. For hard of hearing people this happens all the time. This book is for you—whether you are hearing or hard of hearing! It explains how to communicate with hard of hearing people in one-to-one situations, in groups and meetings, in emergency situations, and in hospitals and nursing homes. When you use the principles given in this book, good things will happen and you will finally be able to have a comfortable chat with a hard of hearing person (38 pages).

When Hearing Loss Ambushes Your Ears—Here's What Happens When Your Hearing Goes on the Fritz ($14.95; eBook $11.95)

Hearing loss often blind-sides you. As a result, your first step should be to learn as much as you can about your hearing loss; then you will be able to cope better. This most interesting book explains how your ears work, the causes of hearing loss, what you can expect to hear with different levels of hearing loss and why you often can't understand what you hear. Lots of audiograms and charts help make things clear. You will also discover a lot of fascinating things about how loud noises damage your ears (88 pages).

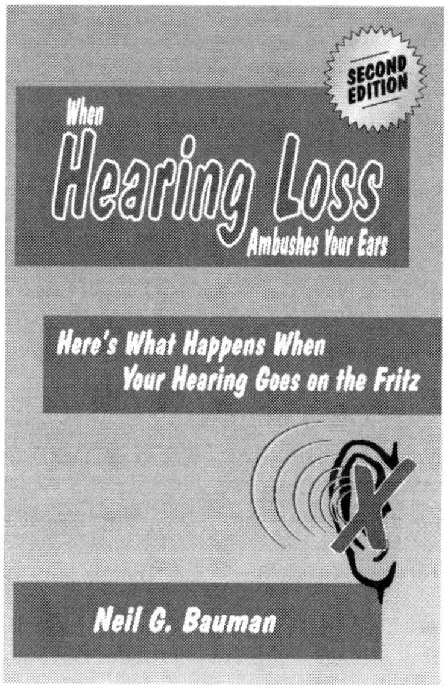

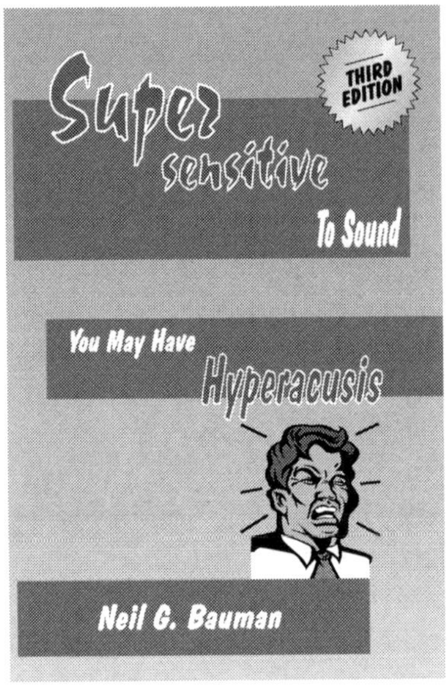

Supersensitive to Sound? You May Have Hyperacusis ($9.95; eBook $7.95)

If some (or all) normal sounds seem so loud they blow your socks off, this is the book you want to read! You don't have to avoid noise or lock yourself away in a soundproof room. Exciting new research on this previously baffling problem reveals what you can do to help bring your hyperacusis under control (42 pages).

Here! Here! You and Your Hearing Loss/You and Your Hearing Aids ($12.95; eBook $10.95)

Part I of this book contains a series of my newspaper articles on hearing loss such as, "Hear Today. Gone Tomorrow?" "Hearing Loss Is Sneaky!" "The Wages of Din Is Deaf!" "When Your Ears Ring..." "Get In My Face Before You Speak!" "How's That Again?" "Being Hard of Hearing Is Hard" "I'm Deaf, Not Daft!" Part II contains articles on hearing aids such as, "You Better Watch Out..." "Before Buying Your First Hearing Aid..." "Please Don't Lock Me Away in Your Drawer" "Good-bye World of Silence!" "Becoming Friends with Your Hearing Aids" "Two's Better Than One!" (56 pages).

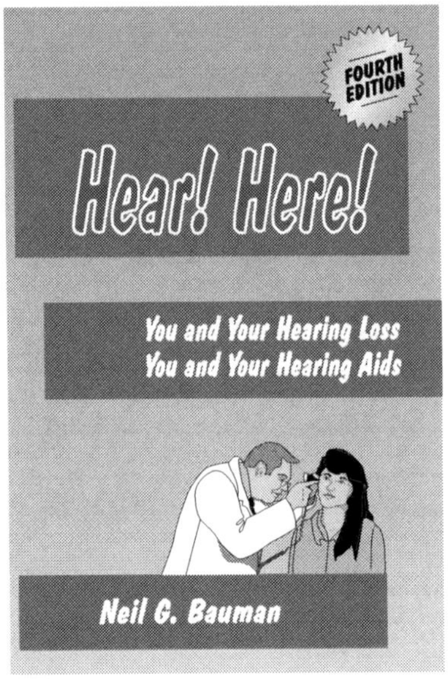

You can order any of the foregoing books/eBooks (plus you can read more than 1,000 helpful articles about hearing loss and related issues) from the

Center for Hearing Loss Help

web site at

http://hearinglosshelp.com

or order them from the address below

Center for Hearing Loss Help

1013 Ridgeway Drive,
Lynden, WA 98264-1057
Phone: (360) 778-1266
FAX: (360) 389-5226
E-mail: info@hearinglosshelp.com
Web site: http://hearinglosshelp.com

Made in the USA
Monee, IL
05 November 2026

67811474R00072